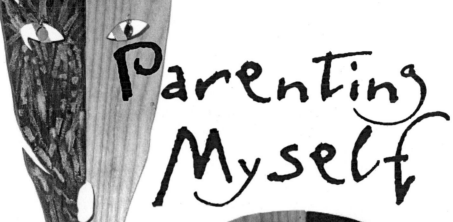

# Parenting Myself

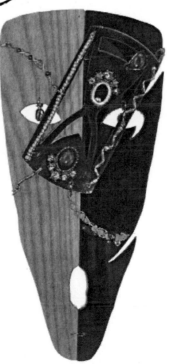

## Recovery from Traumatic Brain Injury

# About *Parenting Myself*

*Parenting Myself: Recovery from Traumatic Brain Injury* by Earlene Ahlquist Chadbourne. $14.95

On August 14, 1990, Earlene Ahlquist Chadbourne went for a casual bicycle ride on a rural road in Saco, Maine. Six days later she woke up in a hospital unable to identify her husband as her husband and incapable of performing many of the skills she had mastered in her former life. All four quadrants of her brain had been injured. Thus began Chadbourne's long healing journey to regain memory and lost skills. Based on the extensive journals the author kept during the recovery process, *Parenting Myself: Recovery from Traumatic Brain Injury* is the story of that journey. For anyone whose sense of identity is woven into what they can do, forgetting long-held skills is much like losing one's self. *Parenting Myself* is the story of skills and a life lost and regained.

**About the Cover:**
Internationally known artists and mask makers Philip and Maria Annal of Winterbound Studio in Grand Isle, Maine, were inspired by the author's story to create this unique depiction of the traumatic brain injury caused by her horrific accident and eventual healing. The hourglass, which adorns the mask and which denotes the time needed for healing, is embellished with gems of malachite and quartz, ancient symbols of brain growth and intelligence. The work clearly conveys the contrast between the damaged self and one that has been lovingly rebuilt.

**To order additional copies:**
Custom Communications, Inc.  or   Kitty Ahlquist Chadbourne
orders@desktoppub.com            www.parentingmyself.com
(207) 286-9295

# Parenting Myself

## Recovery from Traumatic Brain Injury

*E A Chadbourne*

### Earlene Ahlquist Chadbourne

**Custom Communications**

PUBLISHER

Biddeford, Maine

*This volume is dedicated to all who suffer with brain injury and to all the caretakers who accept and encourage the best in those who are injured and do not disparage them for not being the people they used to be. Your friendship is a gift.*

Custom Communications, Inc.
11 Wentworth Street, Biddeford, ME 04005
http://www.desktoppub.com

Library of Congress Cataloging-in-Publication Data
Chadbourne, Earlene Ahlquist.
 Parenting myself : recovery from traumatic brain injury / Earlene Ahlquist Chadbourne.
   p. cm.
Includes bibliographical references.
ISBN 978-1-892168-13-9
1. Chadbourne, Earlene Ahlquist--Mental health. 2. Brain damage--Patients--Maine--Biography. I. Title.

RC387.5.C515 2009
617.4'81044092--dc22
 [B]
                                        2009023694
Printed in the United States of America.

Design, typography, and setup: Custom Communications, Inc.
Photography: © 2009 Deb Wright
Illustrations: Clipart.com, 124, 126
Cover image: © 2009 Philip Annal and Maria Annal
Cover photograph: © 2009 John C. Gold
Cover design: Susan Dudley Gold

1  3  5  6  4  2

# Praise for *Parenting Myself*

"Wow! This story triggers the numerous flashbacks of my own injuries and the aftermaths. Recovering from such an injury is more of a fight than anyone would guess and leaves lasting effects on our lives. Reading this account brings one of similar experiences constantly close to tears because it is so accurate. It needed to be said. Well done."

Kent Verity, USN veteran, retired engineer, TBI survivor

"This is a poignant, honest, and reflective journal of a woman whose perseverance and determination to 'be all she can be' following a traumatic event is a role model for all of us. It stresses the importance of family and the support of friends in the recovery and the importance of faith in the healing process. It shows that finding the 'right' providers/experts is essential."

Meridyth Astrosky, registered/licensed occupational therapist

"Your manuscript brought me to tears of sadness and delight many times. It is wonderful! I could feel your struggle and really couldn't put the story down. Although great strides have been made, there are still so many people who could benefit and find hope and information from your personal account."

Stacy Camire, registered/licensed occupational therapist

"The lessons of your book are useful to veterans and all others inflicted with TBI. But they have much greater range. Others could benefit from the same therapies. Stroke victims have a form of brain injury. The aging process, too, while less acute, affects the brain; many symptoms are the same."

Jim Friedlander, president, Veterans Housing Coalition of Maine

"Your book is an inspiration to me, and your advice is invaluable. As a caregiver to my sister, a TBI patient, I appreciate your honesty in revealing your personal experience. Thanks to you, I am beginning to understand my sister's actions, and I feel that I can see my way to help her. The concrete advice and the 'to do' lists are so very helpful. Watching my sister improve is like watching the hands on a clock, but there is improvement. As you suggested, we are now connected with a nearby TBI center that gives us some respite."

Martin T. Tyler, Captain (Ret.) USN, DDS, MEd, Diplomate ABOM, caregiver of TBI patient

"This is a great resource for traumatic brain injury patients and their caretakers. Very, very helpful, it is filled with practical, down-to-earth advice. It is a compelling story."

Ron Houle, licensed clinical social worker/psychotherapist

"A treasure of a book! A must-read for anyone who has a family member with traumatic brain injury or stroke, and a wonderful guide and comfort for anyone who has suffered through it! I was so touched by this book that I frequently found myself with tears in my eyes.

"In addition to working with patients with TBI, stroke, and chronic pain for forty-plus years, I became a TBI patient myself after a truck rear-ended my car on a California highway in June 2004. For the next two years I struggled to recover from TBI and multiple injuries.

"This special book is a joy and a tribute to optimism and the human spirit. I marveled at the ability of Ms. Chadbourne to put together a treatment path that worked. Part of the unique quality of this book is the wonderful way the author correlates personal experiences with objective knowledge. Medically oriented notes help summarize and add to one's understanding.

"A poignant poem within this book underscores the whole dreadful dilemma: does being an invalid mean that somehow one has become invalid? This book stresses that finding out how to recover what was lost is as important as dealing with the grief and fear that are inevitable. Aside from the soothing matter-of- factness which helps so much in a time of turmoil, this book actively guides the treatment process.

"I cried at the section recounting a Thanksgiving dinner where the author is trying to learn how to cook all over again. The confusion of her sons over whether all this fuss was really necessary brought back my experiences with my three sons, whose support is the only reason I survived at all. Like so many passages in this book, I kept relating it to my own experiences. How I wish this book had been available to us then! "Five years after my accident, I'm back working at the many facets of my life. But my sons and I wish we had had this book to read to help us find the way instead of stumbling constantly. This is an excellent guidebook to those foggy, barely charted corners of the mind that need exploring and a breathe of fresh air when recovering from TBI."

Madeline M. Daniels, Ph.D., licensed clinical and forensic psychologist, author, social activist

"This volume of recovery from traumatic brain injury is both engaging and readable and full of valuable information. Mrs. Chadbourne offers not only a moving portrayal of how she struggled to overcome her injury, but she also highlights the significant ripple effect her injury had on her husband, family, and associates. When a family member suffers from TBI, the entire family is affected. I would urge caretakers and persons who have suffered from brain injuries to read this book."

Michael Brennan, MA, MSW, licensed clinical social worker, former Maine State Senate chair, Joint Standing Committee on Health and Human Services

# Acknowledgments

I am deeply grateful to all who have contributed to the completion of this book. Their encouragement and continued belief that this was an important story to tell kept me trudging along when I might otherwise have given up. I thank my family and friends for being there for me during the trying ordeal of the accident and recovery process and for having the courage to become vulnerable through the publishing of this story for the sake of others' healing.

It has been a daunting task to recreate this story, and I have had to depend on the recollections of many to give a thorough accounting. People in the book have been identified with permission; others have been given pseudonyms to protect their privacy.

Dad, Betty, Ted, Guy, Adam, Deborah, Tania, Dori, Teri, Todd, Lorraine, Barbara, Cindy, Shirley, Debbie, Lorrie, Den, Dory, Roy and Maryllyn, Sue, Harriet and George, Ted and Ruth, Kent, Martin and Mignon, Sallie, Vera, Sharon, Denis, Linda, Stacy, Meridyth, Madeline, Jim, John, and Mike—you each contributed in vital ways to keep me on track and on the path to healing. My medical team with superb care from Maine Medical Center, Dr. Joseph Corbett Jr., Dr. Judy Shedd, Dr. John Knowles, and Dr. James Mancini—each worked seamlessly with the others for my benefit. Dr. Shedd continued the follow-through, always giving me her best.

I can't say thank you enough. May this work become the encouragement to others that you have been to me.

—EAC

# Preface

When my mother sustained a severe brain injury in 1990, little did I know how much that one event would change my life. The entire family struggled to cope with the challenges we had to face as we watched her efforts to regain her health. We did not know how to help. It was frustrating and at times scary.

My mother persevered in the day-to-day campaign she waged on the road to recovery, always encouraging us in the process. I never really knew how much she struggled until I urged her to write her story to help the returning vets and their families who cope with the effects of traumatic brain injury.

My year serving in Iraq brought my mother's situation into focus as I saw firsthand the damage done to my fellow U.S. service members from the improvised explosive devices and other weapons used to target them. I realized that those families were going to have to deal with the same issues my family faced so many years ago after Mom went on a simple bike ride in rural Maine and ended up, hardly recognizable, in a hospital. So I asked her to share her story.

Recent statistics reveal that 320,000 U.S. vets serving in Iraq and Afghanistan are afflicted with TBI. An astounding 1.4 million more people in the civilian population suffer from brain injuries annually. Though incredible progress has been made in the detection and treatment of TBI, the hard work still remains for patients and caretakers in the day-by-day regimen required to take back their lives. This is a job for the marathon runner, not the sprinter. There are no easy fixes.

Families can be devastated by this—ours was. But we healed and are better for the pain, and yours can heal, too. TBI patients can be severely damaged—my mom was. But she grew beyond her injury—and so can you. She'll show you how. To my fellow vets who have brain injuries and to others with TBI, I encourage you to open this book and take the first steps to recovery and your new life.

—Captain Adam R. Cote, Maine Army National Guard, Iraq War veteran

# Contents

# Foreword

THIS MEMOIR WAS WRITTEN primarily for the victims of traumatic brain injury (TBI) and their caregivers. As the numbers of wounded warriors returning from the wars in Iraq and Afghanistan mounted, my heart wept for them, knowing the multiple challenges they would face in their recovery.

And I remembered.

I remembered my own pain, my confusion, my unsteadiness, and even my despair. I remembered wishing something had been written, in language I could understand, by someone who had walked that path before me. There was very little out there; and what was available needed to be dissected and interpreted.

And all I had to guide me was a damaged brain.

We are far more fortunate today. Dedicated professionals have made available a wealth of material to help patients in the twenty-first century. But people with TBI still need a friend who can come alongside and say, "It's okay. I've been down this road before. I'll walk with you."

That is what this book is meant to do. It is designed as a companion, a "big sister" for those traveling the TBI road.

I structured this intimate story with TBI patients in mind. Following many chapters I have included a retrospection and a medical description of the pertinent brain injury. For me, and for many of those with TBI, being able to identify the reasons behind the failures led to a sense of how to get beyond the suffering. That is what this memoir is all about.

So you have traumatic brain injury. It does not have to ruin your life.

# Section I

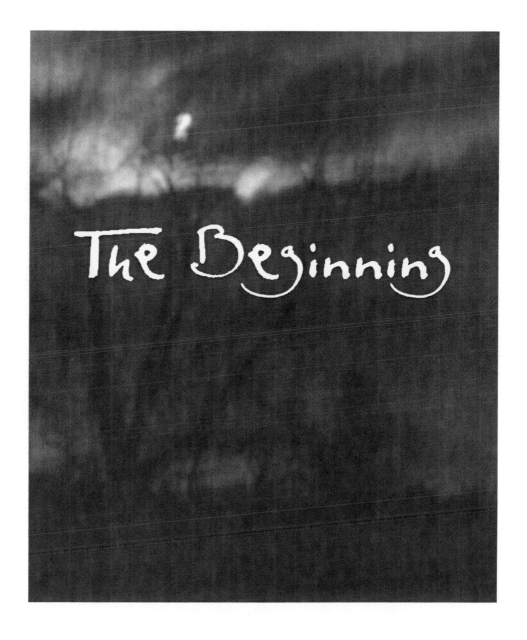

The Beginning

# To Begin Again

I miss the me
I used to be—

In'-va-lid, or
          In-val'-id,
I wonder as I struggle
To learn again
To tie my shoes.

"They keep thinking of my good, in their terms,"
          the old man had said.
"I don't blame them, I only resist them,"*
          he added.

He had reached his angle of repose—
          That fragile balancing point,
          Where life is never
          In-val'-id,
          As it renews in stillness.

*with thanks to Wallace Stegner, *Angle of Repose*

EAC/1990

# 1

# The Accident

ON AUGUST 14, 1990, I awoke to a sunny, beautiful day. Life seemed good again. I had been remarried for eighteen months; my two sons, Guy and Adam, had turned out to be fine young men; and I was beginning to get acquainted with my four step-daughters. On that Tuesday I was looking forward to visiting my cousin Cindy. Since it was such a lovely morning, I thought, "Why not bike to her house?" She lived only three miles from my home in Saco, Maine. To reach her, I had to go through pasture lands in a part of town that tourists on Route One rarely experienced. With some anticipation, I brewed my morning coffee and ate breakfast with my husband, Ted. "I'll be back home to fix lunch," I assured him. (Ted has no kitchen skills!) Then, after cleaning up our breakfast dishes, I walked to the garage, where Ted helped me ready his bike for the trip. Kissing him good-bye, I headed out, promising I'd be home before lunchtime. But . . .

As noon approached and I had not arrived home, Ted began to wonder what had happened. It was not like me to say one thing and do another. He phoned Cindy.

"She never showed up at my house," Cindy told him.

After Ted hung up, Cindy had an unsettling memory—she recalled hearing a report of a bicycle accident on her scanner that morning. Panicky, she phoned the Saco police. The officer who answered the call asked for a description of her cousin before releasing any information about the accident. He said the victim had no identification on her.

Fear seized Cindy as she described me to the police. "She's a small woman with long, blonde hair. Her hands and feet are small, and she has an unusual wedding ring that has a blue stone."

"That's her," the officer said. "We think she suffered a severe head injury. She was taken to Southern Maine Medical Center in Biddeford, but she's at Maine Medical Center now."

Cindy contacted Ted immediately.

After Cindy's rapid-fire call, Ted phoned my dad and my son Guy, who was visiting, to alert them both. They arranged to meet Ted at the hospital. Then Ted phoned his daughter Tania, and she contacted her three sisters.

As he sped along country roads—intent on getting to Maine Medical Center in Portland, a half-hour's drive away—Ted passed my grandmother's familiar white farm house without noticing it. Negotiating a left turn onto another road, he slowed down and saw with horror the blood splattered on the intersection ahead. The terrible sight left him shaking. What condition would I be in when he finally got to Maine Medical Center? Would I even be alive?

With the hospital finally in sight, he found his way blocked by a passing train. It seemed to Ted to be the slowest train in the world. And he was six cars back! In desperation, he shifted into park, left the car idling, and quickly walked to the front of the line. Urgency in his voice, he asked each driver to move out of the way so he could be the first to cross the tracks when the train had passed. Amazingly, they all agreed. The bar finally rose and he raced to the emergency entrance of the hospital.

As soon as Ted entered my room, a shocking image confronted him. I lay unconscious in the hospital bed, blood and spinal fluid draining from my left ear. Cuts covered my body.

Soon my father and Guy arrived, and they, too, were stunned to find me in such critical condition. While Ted dealt with the necessary paper work, Dad and Guy went in to see me. Athletic and twenty-one, Guy had endured many of his own injuries. Driving to the hospital with his grandfather, he had tried to reassure them both that I was not likely to be seriously injured in a bicycle accident. But when he saw the bleeding, unconscious woman, Guy could hardly believe she was his mother. He turned back to the waiting room. There Ted and his grandfather, who had always resembled John Wayne in Guy's mind, were dissolved in tears. Guy had never seen his grandfather weep. The three men huddled on the waiting room couch.

The doctor who had diagnosed me gave them a quick rundown of my condition and what the medical team planned to do in the next few hours. Of most concern—and rapidly endangering my survival—was the swelling in my brain. The brain damage was widespread. It included a concussion in the right front temple area. This concussion had resulted in prefrontal lobe lesions. There was also damage to the temporal lobe and motor cortex in the left part of the brain. In addition, a vital nerve serving the left ear had been severed.

The medical team planned to drill a hole through my skull to try to ease dangerous swelling of the brain and to monitor any new swelling that might occur. If the swelling did not recede within forty-eight hours, a portion of my brain would have to be removed. If I survived the next forty-eight hours, I would have a second chance at life.

My three fellows listened grimly. This was hard news.

My seventeen-year-old son, Adam, still had no idea of my situation. Guy phoned him. Adam, a high-school senior, was just getting out of football practice in Sanford, about forty miles from the medical center. After my divorce from his father, Adam lived with me during the week but attended high school in Sanford. During the summer he worked in Sanford and lived with his father. Guy did not tell his brother how bad things were. He just said, "Mom's had an accident. You've got to come."

Adam arrived an hour and a half later. Like Guy, he was an athlete, and he had sustained his own set of injuries. "A bicycle accident?" he thought. "No real problem." Even his brother's serious expression did not alarm him. But as soon as he entered my cubicle, shock overcame him. He was certain there must be some mistake. That ashen-colored woman lying there with a tube protruding from her forehead could not be his mother.

In the hours and days to come, Ted and the boys—desperate to find something positive to do—became sleuths working with police and doctors to figure out what had happened. The extent of my injuries suggested two separate accidents had occurred, one after the other. Because of the serious hematomas on the left side of my body, they surmised that I had been hit by a car first and had lain in the road for several hours before getting back on the bike.

No one ever reported such an incident to the police. The second accident, however, had two witnesses who saw me riding unsteadily down a hill ahead of their car. The driver put his brakes on, refusing to pass me. He commented to his wife, "We'd better wait. She looks like she's having trouble."

They reported that the front wheel of my bicycle wobbled as I tried to control the handlebars. The hapless couple watched in horror as, still heading downhill, I fell forward over the handlebars and landed on my head. The woman, a licensed practical nurse, ministered to me as best she could while her husband went to a nearby house to call the police and an ambulance.

The officer who reported to the scene made a succinct report of the situation as she found it:

> On Tues., 08/14/90 at 1340 hrs., this officer was dispatched to the intersection of Heath & Mc-Kenney Road in ref. to a bicyclist being injured. Saco Rescue responding as well. Upon arrival, a female was observed laying face down on the pavement in the middle of the intersection of McKenney and Heath Roads. A bicycle was lying on the pavement close by. Female was bleeding from the head and ear area. A female witness, identifying herself as an LPN, was holding a towel to the injured female's head. Saco Rescue arrived a few seconds after this officer and took over caring for the injured female. Female was unable to tell us her name or any information and was conscious but not coherent upon officer's arrival. This officer spoke to two witnesses.

While reading the report, Ted and Dad recalled that I had always ridden bikes with foot brakes. Ted's bike, which was new to me, had hand brakes. Had I gripped the brakes too tightly and catapulted over the handlebars when the bike stopped suddenly? That seemed plausible for the second accident, but what about the first? Had I been hit by a driver who had sped off, leaving me bleeding and too dazed to know what I was doing when I got back on the bike? Could someone have left me to die?

The family waited in agony as each hour crept by. Lorraine, my younger half-sister and Tania, Ted's daughter, took turns washing blood out of my hair and gently combing it during their five-minute visits to my bedside. Thanks to them, I was not shaved bald. Despite all their efforts and concern, I remained in a coma. The next forty-eight hours were critical. Would the swelling in my brain stop in time? Would a portion of my brain have to be removed? How would I fare then? Would I survive? And if I did, who would I be?

# 2

# In the Hospital

*At the close of WW I, thousands of shell-shocked veterans in France suffered from amnesia. The lack of identification tags complicated the situation. Eventually French authorities brought the soldiers to a great gathering at a large plaza in Paris. One by one the confused soldiers walked to the platform and simply said, "Won't someone please tell me who I am?"*

SIX DAYS AFTER THE ACCIDENT I awoke in a room that was not my own. The room, obviously in a hospital, had green walls, and the sun shone through the windows. What was I doing there?

"Can you tell me your name?" asked a friendly but unfamiliar voice. It was a woman's voice.

"Earlene," I replied. "Who are you?" I focused on the pleasant voice. It came from a brunette standing next to my bed smiling.

"Pam," she said. "I'm your nurse. You are at Maine Medical Center. You were in a bicycle accident. You've injured your head."

After the crucial forty-eight hours had passed, doctors had told the family that I was out of critical condition and could be moved to a room in the special care unit. They could not yet determine, however, the extent of brain injury.

How long had I been here? I wondered, looking around. I saw the tubes attached to both of my arms and the safety rails on each side of the bed. I was too weak and confused to observe more. Pam maneuvered efficiently about the bed doing her work. What was going on?

Then I saw my father standing at the end of my bed, smiling. I felt safer.

"Kits," Dad started to say. Pam gestured with her hand, and he stopped.

"Tell me your name again, your full name," Pam commanded.

"Earlene Ahlquist."

"And who is this man?"

"Dad."

"What is his name?"

"Earle Ahlquist."

"And do you have another name?"

"Kitty or Kits."

"And where are you?"

"The hospital."

Then, from somewhere, Ted approached the bed and reached for my hand.

"And who is this?"

"Ted."

"Ted who?"

"Ted Chadbourne," I replied.

"And who is he?"

"My cousin," I said, and, at that moment, I was overcome with fatigue and fell back to sleep.

Ted gulped and held his breath.

Dad reached over and patted him on the shoulder, "It will come, Ted. You were a cousin long before you became a husband. It will come." Ted let his breath out and nodded.

A steady stream of relatives and friends visited me at the hospital, but I don't have many memories of that time. Mostly I remember my father being there, steadfast and loving. I remember Ted being there only occasionally, yet I have been told that he visited every day. Guy and Adam were there daily, too, but I don't remember that. I remember only my father.

My father and I have always had a special relationship. After my mother committed suicide when I was sixteen, we went through that very dark time together. The same unique bond that often connects people who share traumatic experiences deepened our father-daughter relationship. Throughout my life, in my dark times, while struggling with life itself and with my own identity as a person, I always turned to my father.

This was a hard time for Ted. I had been identifying myself to the nurses as Earlene Ahlquist, my maiden name, not Earlene Ahlquist Chadbourne, the name I had been using as Ted's wife for the last eighteen months. When asked who Ted was, I continued to answer that he was my cousin, and he was. We were fifth cousins, twice removed, having met at a family reunion several years earlier.

When a cousin asked Ted how he was doing through all this stress, he simply replied, "If I lost my ability to know people, if I had Alzheimer's, I know Kitty would still be there for me. So, I'll be here for her. We will get past this."

Nurses kept waking me so that I would not fall back into a deeper coma. I responded little to their prompts. When I did respond, it was only for a brief moment before I drifted back into what seemed to be a perpetual sleep. Everyone wanted me to regain consciousness and speak more than a few words. But that would not be for a while. My father urged patience. One day when Dad was at my bedside, a nurse asked me the date of my birthday.

"April 8, 1949," I said, matter-of-factly. The constant questions had become tedious. The nurse looked at her clipboard. The "right" date, clearly written on the chart, was not April 8. She shook her head.

"What's the matter?" asked my dad, who knew my birthday was April 8 as well as he knew anything.

"She's confused about her birthday again," the nurse said.

"But she's not. She was born on April 8, 1949!"

Thus ended a misunderstanding that had begun when Ted rushed to my side that first day. Hospital officials had asked him for information about me. In his panic, he had written the birth date of his ex-wife! No wonder I kept giving the "wrong" answer!

I recall at some point Dad and Ted standing in the room when the nurse came quizzing me.

"Your name?"

"Earlene Ahlquist Chadbourne," I said as if that were what I had been saying all along.

Ted smiled. A twinkle came to Dad's eye. The nurse grinned.

"What was I usually called?"

"Kitty."

"When was I born?"

" April 8, 1949."

"Where?"

"Portland, Maine."

"Where are you?"

"In the hospital."

"Why are you in the hospital?"

"Bicycle accident."

"Do you realize you had a serious brain injury?"

"Yes."

"Are you scared?"

"No." This was more promising. Perhaps I would get better after all.

\* \* \* \* \*

While I recognized my father from the beginning, my response to Ted, Guy, Adam, and Ted's daughters was much more muted. I used each person's correct name, but I gave little indication that I knew what role they played in my life. When they spoke, I barely responded at all. My sons had always been assured of my love for them, but my lack of response hurt them. (Years later, Adam told me that my flat response to him made him question the depth of our seemingly close relationship.)

Were they being phased out of my life, Guy and Adam continued to ask themselves, to make more time for my new husband? Because visitations were kept to five to ten minutes at first and to one person at a time, Guy and Adam did not witness my lack of response to Ted and others. They did not know that everyone except Dad existed in the same shadowy state in my mind.

\* \* \* \* \*

Dad was one of the few Marines to survive Iwo Jima. His drill sergeant always told him that, when he did not think he could do any more, he should remember that he had used only one-fifth of his resources; four-fifths were still in reserve. How many times had Dad told me this! "It's not just my drill sergeant," he would declare. "Even scientists say that humans use only one tenth of their brain power."

As I continued to fight my way to consciousness, I figured I had four-fifths of my reserves and nine-tenths of my brain left. It all added up to enough brain power to function and perhaps even to grow in the future. My math may have been faulty, but my attitude was right-on.

I would have to get better! That's all there was to it.

Miraculously, I had broken no bones and had damaged no major organs, except my brain. My brain! And no one knew the extent of that damage. I would just have to wait and see.

On August 20, after many CAT scans, the one-inch shunt that monitored swelling in the brain was removed from my head. Later, after I woke up, the intravenous tubes were also taken away, and I began to eat regular food. I could walk with aid, and I could speak haltingly.

After I had been at Maine Medical Center for ten days, neurosurgeon Joseph Corbett; Judy Shedd, my primary care physician; and audiology specialist John Knowles began talking of sending me home. The medical staff scheduled visiting nurses to help me on the medical side, and I would meet weekly with the team of doctors monitoring my recovery. No one addressed who would handle the details of cooking and housekeeping. I had no idea how we would manage, but I was eager to go home and was sure we would find a way.

Doctors supplied me with Dilantin for seizures, Darvocet for moderate pain, Valium for anxiety, and Extra-Strength Tylenol for mild pain. On August 27, 1990, I left the hospital and headed home to begin my new life.

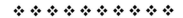

*In Retrospect:*

Tears well up even now, almost twenty years later, when my family reflects on those frightening days in the middle of August 1990 when I hung between life and death.

Those days were difficult, but the days that followed were tougher still. I went home without any preparation for or understanding of what I faced as a person with traumatic brain injury. There were no trauma centers in the region then, and my family and I had no access to counselors trained specifically in brain trauma issues. We received none of the emotional and psychological support so crucial in dealing with brain injuries.

We desperately needed someone to help us all understand our new roles and responsibilities. Without a skilled counselor, we pulled apart, not knowing how to cope with my condition. Ted and the boys did not understand the nature of my injury and had no one to explain my symptoms and advise them on how to respond. They misinterpreted my lack of interest as rejection and reacted by becoming remote.

In some ways, my father provided guidance. His background as an Iwo Jima survivor and the yearlong recovery process he himself had undergone after that ordeal gave him an empathetic perspective. Consequently, he looked for small areas of progress in my cognitive responses and gave me hope by pointing these out to me. He urged Ted and the boys to be patient and to encourage me as much as they could.

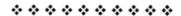

*Medical Description:*

Acquired Brain Injury (ABI) is a general term which includes stroke, aneurism, and traumatic brain injury. TBI is described as an "insult" to the brain. It is not degenerative or congenital, though the diminished and altered state of consciousness has often been compared to that of stroke victims or Alzheimer's patients.

There are two basic types of brain injury, closed head injury (CHI) and open head injury (OHI). I sustained a closed head injury, which included a skull fracture at the base of the brain. Open head injuries are caused by bullets or other penetrating objects. The more common closed head injuries are caused by rapid movements of the head during which the brain is whipped back and forth inside the skull. This often occurs during automobile accidents or severe falls. The effect on the brain inside the skull is catastrophic. The rapid movement pulls apart or stretches the nerve fibers (called axons). This breaks connections between different parts of the brain. Brain contusions (bruises) can result if the injury affects the frontal parts of the brain (which help control behavior and emotions). In most cases, blood vessels rupture as a by-product of the blow, causing a blood clot (hematoma), which can put added pressure on the brain.

I experienced a "contra-coup effect," in which both the site of the injury and the opposite area are injured when the brain bounces back and forth in the skull. As a result, this diffused the injury into many different parts of the brain. Frontal and back damage occurred as well as damage to the left and right sides of the brain (hemispheres).

Dr. Joseph Corbett Jr. summarized my injury on the discharge papers:

> **History of Present Illness:** Earlene Chadbourne is a 40-year-old woman who was in a bike accident and was thrown onto asphalt. She was following commands on arrival at Maine Medical Center. She was leaking cerebrospinal fluid from the left ear. She was moving her arms and legs symmetrically. Pupils were equal and reactive. A CAT scan showed a right temporal lobe contusion with blood in the sulci. There was a smaller contusion on the left side. A C-spine was within normal limits. The patient was intubated on arrival and had to remain intubated and

required sedation. Because she was agitated and confused, it was decided to place an intracranial pressure sensor. This was done and the intracranial pressure has remained low. She was able to be extubated and was transferred to the floor. Her scalp laceration was closed. She had contusions in several places and a moderately sized hematoma on the left thigh. The cerebrospinal fluid leak stopped and there were no episodes of meningitis. Her hearing was somewhat decreased and she was evaluated by Dr. Knowles, who recommended a follow-up visit in the office for definitive evaluation. Mrs. Chadbourne's blood pressure was transiently elevated and this responded well to Nifedipine, both p.o. and sublingually, and Anallopril. By the discharge, her systolic and diastolic blood pressure had improved and the dosages were decreased prior to discharge. She will arrange to have primary care evaluation and further evaluation of her need for blood pressure medication. Her Decadron was able to be tapered and this was discontinued. She was maintained on Dilantin and did not have evidence of seizures. She was alert and oriented but had slight decrease in short-term memory and a slight decrease in inhibitions. She is to return to the office in two weeks and will have a head CAT scan without contrast. The diagnoses listed: 1. post head injury, temporal lobe contusions 2. left otorrhea, 3. left hematoma.

*Medical Definitions:*

CAT scan, also called C-T scan—computed tomography, a computerized sensing device that gathers digital data or images of an organ or area of the body.

contusion—bruise.

C-spine—portion of the spine in the cervix, or neck.

diastolic blood pressure—second and lower measurement recording the force of blood as the heart is filling before the next beat.

extubated—removal of tube from the body.

hematoma—a localized swelling filled with blood resulting from a break in a blood vessel.

intubated—insertion of tube into the body.

intracranial pressure sensor—a device placed inside the head which senses the pressure inside the brain cavity and sends its measurement to a recording device.

motor cortex— regions of the brain that plan, control, and execute voluntary motor functions.

otorrhea—discharge from the ear.

p.o.—post-operative; following surgery.

post head injury—damage that occurs after the accident or event.

sub-lingually—below or beneath the tongue.

sulci—fissure between two convolutions (irregular ridges) in the brain.

systolic blood pressure—first and higher measurement recording the peak force of blood as it is being pumped by the heart.

temporal lobes—two sections of the brain located on both sides of head above the ears, involved with memory, emotion, hearing, and language.

# 3

# Home Again

DEN AND DORY HOWARD-CORRIN, dear friends, came to the hospital the Monday I was discharged. They met Ted and helped bring me home. Ted had rented a walker from the local pharmacy and had filled all my prescriptions. The two men rode in the front seats, and Dory sat beside me in the back.

On the way to our home in Saco, I began to feel motion sickness. (When I was a child, I had often experienced motion sickness while riding.) As waves of dizziness and faintness washed over me, the car continued to jostle me. My poor brain was not up for the ride! The half-hour drive that I had taken so many times before seemed that day to last forever.

Hospital evaluators had judged our home, a fifteen-year-old Cape Cod, to be sufficiently accessible for a person in my condition. The master bedroom had a full bath nearby. Although our bedroom was on the second level, the stairs leading up to it had safety rails. A year earlier we had refinished the basement into a family room with an adjacent hot tub room. (I would be very grateful for the hot tub later to ease the pain from the massive hematomas remaining on my left thigh.)

That summer Guy and Adam worked thirty miles away in

Sanford and stayed with their father, who had a home there. Ted's older daughters, Deborah, Tania, and Dori, lived on their own. His youngest, Teri, spent every other weekend with us. There would be no busy flurry of people constantly in flux or rambunctious pets. My gray cat, Shadow, was gentle-natured and soothing. It was going to be good to get home.

As soon as we arrived at the house, Dory started preparing lunch. In no time she had a meal ready. It was my first meal at home since the accident, almost two weeks ago. I felt utterly blessed—and exhausted!

After lunch, I did not linger. I wanted very much to lie down. Dory helped me to the bedroom. To my great relief, I had no problem climbing the stairs with her gentle hand guiding me. Once in the bedroom, I lay down, overcome with exhaustion and feeling as if I had just fought a battle.

Before leaving, Dory checked our refrigerator, filled with meals prepared for us by friends and family members. Dory set to work marking everything with explicit directions for Ted, who had little experience as a cook. While she worked, Den and Ted wrote our schedule of upcoming doctors' appointments on the calendar.

Having done what they could, Den and Dory headed home, promising to call the next day. I drifted into sleep.

My convalescence at home had begun.

* * * * *

Ted's cousin, Lorrie, who was a nurse, lived nearby with her husband, John. Later in the week she came to remove the stitches from my basal skull fracture. I came downstairs for the procedure. Lorrie seated me at the dining room table, where the light was brightest.

"Tip your head, Kitty," she said, and I obeyed.

Gently, Lorrie pulled my long hair away from the stitches.

John had come, too, and he kindly tried to distract me as Lorrie carefully removed the stitches that extended several inches around the back and left side of my skull. Though she had a gentle touch, the procedure hurt, and I winced.

"Kitty, knock, knock," John immediately called out.

I did not answer him as Lorrie continued to remove the stitches.

"Come on, Kitty, say 'Who's there?'"

"Who's there?"

"Misses."

Another pause and then John said, "Ask 'Misses who?'"

"Misses who?"

"Mississippi."

I smiled. At least, he was trying, and I appreciated that.

John laughed. Encouraged now, he launched into another "knock, knock" joke.

"Who's there?" I asked.

"Butter."

"Butter who?"

"Butterfly."

I giggled. The stitches were out.

# 4

# Settling In

FOR A FULL WEEK after I returned home, we ate plentifully from the meals that family and friends had generously provided us. For this bounty I was very grateful because Ted had no idea how to cook. He managed to open a Campbell's soup can and heat the contents. He could prepare himself a bowl of Cheerios. But that was pretty much it. He could not even brew coffee and thought doughnuts were one of the four major food groups.

Each night during that first week Ted fetched a prepared meal from the refrigerator and microwaved it according to Dory's directions. After we had eaten, he loaded our dishes into the dishwasher. I noticed his pride as he said, "The girls taught me how to run the dishwasher while you were in the hospital."

"How's that?" I asked.

"Well," Ted admitted. "We have a very clean floor because originally I used the liquid detergent in the dishwasher. Bubbles all over the floor!" He smiled, laughing at himself and the recollection. "Then I was instructed in the proper detergent to use. I never knew things could be so complicated! I sure am glad you're home to straighten things out. Yes, they also showed me how to run the clothes washer. But I still haven't figured out how you hang clothes on the clothesline so neatly. I admire your determination to save energy, but I don't see how I'll ever be able to hang clothes like you do."

"I think we can use the dryer for a while," I replied. Just thinking about carrying a basket of clothes outside and bending down to retrieve a shirt and then stretching to pin it on the line made me dizzy.

Incredibly, Ted turned down offers of help, certain, in spite of an emptying refrigerator and an increasingly untidy house, that we didn't need to trouble anyone. Because I could now speak haltingly and read slowly, everyone presumed that I was bouncing back and would continue to do so. When Ted said we didn't need help, friends and family backed away. No doubt, Ted wanted to reestablish the sense of "just the two of us" before Adam joined us at the start of the school year. He would be staying in our home and driving to high school in Sanford.

\* \* \* \* \*

Later in the week of my return home, I prepared for my first medical appointment, scheduled for Friday, August 31, with Judy Shedd, my osteopathic physician. Dr. Shedd had seen me through a series of minor skiing accidents in the past, and we had developed a wonderful rapport. Her office in North Bridgton is about an hour's drive northwest of our home. While I looked forward to seeing her, I dreaded the ride.

Ted drove carefully, curbing his usual tendency to speed. Even so, every bump jarred me and seemed to send my brain rattling. The motion sickness that had so disturbed me on the drive from Portland three days earlier was even worse on this trip. Nausea and faintness assaulted me. I hated the thought of having to ride back home again over that rolling terrain with its curves and bumps.

As soon as I walked into the waiting room, Dr. Shedd greeted me with a warm smile, saying, "Kitty, already you look better than in the hospital. We're planning for your recovery." She laughed her hearty laugh. "Come into the office. I'm going to ask my associate, Dr. James Jealous, to check you over first. He's very experienced in cranial problems."

Dr. Shedd helped me onto the examining table. I lay on my back while Dr. Jealous ran his hands gently over my skull. He spoke to Dr. Shedd as he observed my responses to his touch. They talked in "doctor-speak," which I did not understand. I closed my eyes and relaxed. A moment later, Dr. Shedd examined my head and spine in a similar manner.

After Dr. Jealous left the room, I asked, "When I came in, you said that I looked better than in the hospital. I don't remember your being there."

"Oh yes," she said. "I saw you several times. I conferred with Dr. Corbett, the hospital's neurosurgeon, and Dr. Knowles, who will handle the hearing problems. I believe you are scheduled to see him soon. "

"I don't remember, but I think Ted has appointments written on the calendar."

Dr. Shedd smiled reassuringly. "Kitty, the way this brain injury works is that as your fractured skull heals, parts of your brain are sort of on sabbatical. We'll nudge it along as things start to heal and fall back into place. I will use cranial manipulation, osteopathy, and homeopathic remedies because of your high sensitivity to many prescription drugs—though I reserve the right to use drugs if necessary. We will meet weekly. I want you to note the things you are having trouble doing and let me know every week. I want you to give your body permission to heal by not demanding too much from it. That means about twelve hours of sleep a night and naps if you need it in between."

I smiled and nodded, reassured by her words.

"Call me if there are any problems," she said.

I left feeling I was in good hands. It helped soothe the rough ride home. Fortunately, the journey was less arduous than the earlier one. Ted chose a route with flatter terrain for the return trip. Terrain and speed, it seemed, affected my nausea.

\* \* \* \* \*

By the next week, in early September, Ted and I had run out of prepared food. I was hungry. I resolved to make a meal. I called for Ted, who was downstairs at his computer. He didn't hear me.

Determined that I could get down to the kitchen alone, I eased myself cautiously out of bed. Steadying myself by fingering the walls, I arrived at the stairs. So many steps—thirteen in all! Walking upstairs had not been difficult, but I had not yet tried to walk down the stairs alone. Clinging to the railing, I began my descent. With each step, I felt real terror, certain I would fall forward. But I continued, pausing on every stair. Very slowly, I reached the first floor—safely. Turning left and taking careful steps, I made my way through the dining room to the kitchen.

I reached for my handwritten recipe book. It contained my favorites, my comfort food, and that day I wanted comfort. With care, I scanned the recipes and chose one. Then, crossing to the cupboard, I pulled the ingredients I would need and placed them on the counter.

For a moment I stood and looked at the items stacked before me. Then I realized I had no clue what to do with the strange assortment I had just assembled. What was going on here? Was someone playing a cruel game of bait and switch? Surely I should be able to follow my own recipes. I had cooked since early childhood. I couldn't imagine that I would not be able to do something I had done easily for so long.

I reached for the phone to call my Aunt Barbara for help. "What am I supposed to do with the ingredients?" I asked. "What does 'temperature' mean? What about the different measurements, and how are they mixed? Why do so many recipes just list the ingredients with no description of how to mix them? When directions call for a 'prepared pan,' what does that mean?"

"Mimi and I will be right up," Aunt Barb replied. Soon she and Mimi, my eighty-two-year-old grandmother, stood in the kitchen with me as we made a meal together. Meatloaf, scalloped potatoes, and green beans. Ted set the table, and we devoured the meal. We even had enough leftovers for Adam when he arrived home from football practice. I was enormously grateful for the help. Even so, I thought, that was only one meal. I have a whole lifetime of meals in front of me.

After Barb and Mimi left, I looked at the kitchen tools, my grandmother's old bowls, the familiar recipes from my childhood, the wooden spoons, the ingredients. They all sat there like an orchestra that had lost its maestro, confused players gazing with blank faces at the empty spot their leader had once occupied. For now and for who knew how far into the future, there would be no aroma of delicious foods cooking at my house, no rattle of pots and pans, no satisfaction at the dinner table.

Ted worked constantly at his computer, focused on the task of the moment. Hunger pangs did not seem to signal him of impending mealtime, but I certainly felt them. Day followed day. Ted presumed that I, who had once been a good cook, would continue to prepare our meals as before. But kitchen chores defeated me, at least for the time being.

"Are you hungry?" I asked him when the hunger pangs became insistent.

His standard reply would be "No thanks." But then he would see the look on my face or detect something in my voice or the shakiness that signals an onset of a hypoglycemic attack, which lack of food triggers in me.

"Let's go out to eat." Ted would say, his usual solution.

The first year after my accident we ate frequently at a little diner near our house. Mimi went through her simpler recipes and wrote step-by-step instructions on how to prepare them. Even with that, I had a difficult time cooking the simplest meals. When we ate at home, we depended a lot on frozen dinners.

# Section II

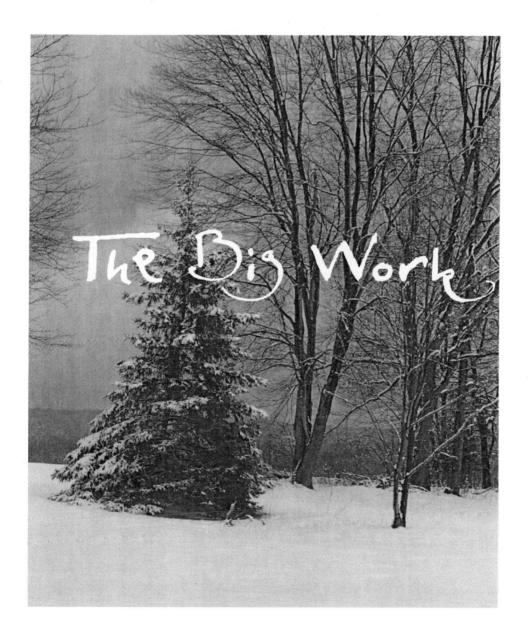

The Big Work

## Shadows

I have a shadow
   it's my dark,  reprobate,  unseemly side—
   the times I'm Angry,
   the times I Shock myself with my thoughts
and wonder—what Nasty Stranger dwells within me,
   sharing my voice and gait

It's my Shadow,  just speaking up.

But sh—sh—sh—it's a Secret,
   Uncovered by my pen as I sketched—
   Changing flat paper to a scene of depth
To have No Shadow
   Is to Not Exist
        Under the Sun.
So  I draw,  I  paint,  I write
   With Shadows
        To be Real.

EAC/1991

# 5

# In Good Hands

A NOTE FROM MY JOURNAL, September 5, 1990:
> *I am so very thankful that I am on track with Judy Shedd. But there's so much wrong with me. I definitely need more than one physician. This hearing, or rather non-hearing, stuff can be very confusing. For instance, a phone call came in while I was resting. Because my left leg is still so sore and swollen, I have been resting on my right side, so the ear with the broken eardrum was to the room. I heard a man's voice leaving a message. I could not distinguish the words. I thought it was Ted's father. He's almost ninety and speaks with a very garbled voice and so is hard to understand. Soon, Ted was nudging me and wanting to hand me the phone. I eased myself up and then held the phone to my good ear, expecting to speak to Ted's dad. I was surprised to hear Adam on the other end of the line. I couldn't recognize my own son's voice.*

My hearing loss disturbed me in those first weeks home. Would this loss be permanent or would I be able to regain my hearing? Fortunately, the week after seeing Dr. Shedd, I had an appointment in Portland on September 6 with Dr. John Knowles, a hearing specialist. I felt certain he would answer my questions and help me to heal. I did not remember Dr. Knowles's examination of my ear while I was hospitalized. Even so, I knew he had gathered information about me and would be ready to help me regain my hearing.

Ted and I had prepared questions and eagerly awaited guidance from the doctor. I had not, however, been looking forward to riding to his Portland office. It proved less difficult than the trip to Bridgton the previous week.

"Was it because the road was straighter and flatter?" I asked Dr. Knowles as we sat with him in his Portland office. He agreed that the smoother terrain probably made the trip easier for me. He said I could use my vision to counter my constant vertigo and general motion sickness. "Focus your eyes on a nonmoving object," he suggested.

He provided other much-needed tips on combatting dizziness and improving balance. I learned from him that if I slid my foot along the floor or pavement, never totally balancing on one foot or the other, my confidence in walking would slowly resume. "You will probably need a cane for a long while yet," he said, "but you might not have to cling to walls as much as you have been."

I learned, too, that my feet sensed vibration, which could also lead to a heightened sense of dizziness. "Avoid escalators and be aware you may feel dizzy even in elevators," he said. Again, he repeated the mantra I would adopt as my own: "Focus your eyes on a nonmoving object."

Dr. Knowles explained the extent of my hearing loss and its effect on other areas. In the early appointments I understood only portions of what he said. I underwent my first audiogram that day. The test, which measured my hearing loss, left me incredibly tired and confused. The headphone I had to wear hurt my head, which was still swollen from the accident. I wanted to cry. Later I would undergo other audiograms, less difficult as I healed, and several speech therapy discrimination tests.

The basal skull fracture I suffered had broken my eardrum and severed a primary nerve leading to my left ear. As a result, I had a substantial hearing loss on my left side, but its extent could not yet be determined until the swelling subsided. I would see Dr. Knowles for a follow-up appointment October 4, followed by a series of tests on November 1. After that I would see the specialist every six months for the next year.

Driving home, tired from the tests, I contemplated all that I had lost since August 14, the last day of my old life. That existence seemed so far removed. Yet the future seemed more than I could comprehend.

I focused on thinking only of the next moment, the next hour—the next immediate thing—like food! We stopped at the grocery on our way home, and Ted went to the frozen food section and picked up a few meals to microwave.

\* \* \* \* \*

For the next nine months Judy Shedd and I met weekly to work through the many complications I faced during my recovery. As a physician, Dr. Shedd took a holistic approach to health care. Together we dealt with each challenge and addressed each of my needs. She actively sought out treatments and approaches that might benefit me. She became my cheerleader, guide, resource person, and friend as well as my physician.

As I slowly recovered and attempted to reclaim portions of my former life, I discovered new areas that gave me trouble. Dr. Shedd administered cranial manipulation treatment, while we discussed the most recent challenge. She offered suggestions on how to cope with the problems. I walked into her office with a list and out with a list.

We celebrated when my health had improved enough to stretch my appointments to every two weeks. Even after almost twenty years, however, I still see Dr. Shedd at least once a month. Stress causes my spinal column and head to become painfully rigid, which results in painful headaches and a return of regressive symptoms.

I met with Dr. Joseph Corbett Jr. twice after coming home from the hospital for routine follow-up appointments. Dr. Corbett checked my reflexes and balance and sent his reports to Dr. Shedd, who remained my primary care physician. Within six months I no longer needed his services.

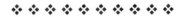

*Medical Description:*

Impairments resulting from ABI/TBI (acquired/traumatic brain injury) fall into three main categories:

**Cognitive Impairments:** short- and long-term memory deficits, slowness of thinking, difficulty in maintaining attention and concentration, impairments of perception, communication, reading and writing skills, reasoning, organization, problem solving, planning, information processing, sequencing, and judgment.

**Physical Impairments:** speech, vision, hearing, and other sensory impairments (loss of smell and taste), headaches, lack of coordination, spasticity of muscles (paralysis of one or both sides), seizure disorders, problems with sleep and balance.

**Psycho-Social, Behavioral, and Emotional Impairments:** fatigue, mood swings, denial, anxiety, depression, self-centeredness, lowered self-esteem, sexual dysfunction, restlessness, lack of motivation, inability to self-monitor, difficulty with emotional control and anger management, inability to cope, agitation, excessive laughing or crying, difficulty in relating to others.

I exhibited impairments of all three types. My cognitive impairments included all the areas mentioned above to some degree. Among my physical impairments were problems with speech, vision, and hearing, headaches, and lack of coordination. The psycho-social impairments included anxiety, depression, and difficulty with emotional control.

# 6

# "What's That You Say?"

I HAD PRESUMED that my loss of hearing was the result of a broken eardrum and a severed nerve, but Dr. Knowles helped me to understand that it was more complicated than that. The injuries done to the temporal lobes, the brain stem, and the cerebellum had resulted in a variety of impairments.

Among the problems I faced were vertigo including nausea, loss of balance, difficulties with movement, and disorganization. These all related to brain stem damage. The severing of the eighth nerve resulted in hearing loss. Injury to the cerebellum interfered with the ability to move rapidly and to coordinate fine movements as well as causing dizziness and slurred speech.

I knew that my hearing would never totally come back, but I began to see progress in other areas. By November 1990, I still walked cautiously with a cane, but I no longer steadied myself by fingering the walls with my other hand.

Motion sickness became less of a problem. By fixing my eyes on the hood medallion of Ted's car as Dr. Knowles had suggested, I no longer felt the waves of nausea that had washed over me before whenever I had to ride anywhere. By the time I underwent the second set of audiogram tests in early November, the swelling of my head had subsided considerably. It no longer hurt when I put on the headphones.

"You have about 11 percent hearing in your left ear but your right ear is generally very good," Dr. Knowles informed me after the second round of tests.

Unfortunately, the little hearing I had in my left ear amplified and distorted all other sounds, especially those in upper frequencies. Children's high-pitched voices echoed loudly in my ear. Even when background noise seemed muted to everyone else, I heard the rushing sound produced by a shell held to one's ear. I heard the reverberating ocean everywhere. This noise made it difficult for me to concentrate and to discriminate other sounds.

With my hearing impairment, I had become a great lover of quiet. Yet even with silence, there was no real quiet for me. To resolve the problem, Dr. Knowles formed a putty block that I could insert in my left ear. It muffled extraneous noises and gave my right ear a chance to hear correctly.

I left the doctor's office full of hope. To celebrate what felt like a good day, Ted and I decided to dine at a local gourmet restaurant for an early supper of superb French cuisine. We had frequented the establishment on many special occasions and always enjoyed it.

I carefully made my way to the designated table in the cozy, old-world dining spot. Determined to appear "normal," I followed Dr. Knowles's advice as I fixed my eyes on an upright beam ahead and tried to ignore the unsteadiness that swept over me when I walked over the uneven floor boards. I breathed a sigh of relief when I sat down opposite Ted. A waiter handed us menus as a server poured chilled water into our goblets. I relaxed into the chair, smoothed the white linen tablecloth, and admired the fresh flowers set before us. Eagerly, I opened the menu and stared at it, stunned.

Finally I asked Ted, " Did I used to read this menu?"

"Oh, yes," Ted replied. "You're my translator. I don't read French, you do."

Not one word of French made sense to me. Two and a half months after the accident, I realized I had lost my ability to read, write, and speak French!

The loss shocked me. What more had I lost that I had not yet realized? I hardly recall the exquisite morsels we consumed that evening at our "celebration." Numbed by the latest revelation of loss, I wondered how long a list I would have for Dr. Shedd on my next visit.

# 7

# Words, Words, and More Words

A NOTE FROM MY JOURNAL, October 10, 1990:

> *It happened again yesterday when Ted and I went to the diner for lunch. Ralph came by and struck up a conversation. I wanted so much to say something. Ralph and Ted waited expectantly for me to reply, but the words I needed had run from me again. Dr. Corbett had warned us of this. Why do I feel like I've been robbed! It makes me look like a simpleton—maybe that's what I've become. Hold on, Girl—you would have objected if either Guy or Adam had used the word "simpleton"—and you, as mother, would have sat them down and talked about that. Learn from having been a good mother to your sons—learn to nurture yourself! Lots of perfectly good words reside in dictionaries—so nurture assignment number one: go find some words, positive ones!*

Following the accident, I noticed I forgot words. I started a sentence and the next word I needed simply vanished. It was not merely a case of using inappropriate words, though I have certainly done that. It was rather like going shopping, putting the groceries away, then going to the cupboard and finding it empty. I had a cupboard full of words, and then I did not.

To counter the missing-word problem, I kept a thesaurus and a dictionary next to my bed. I also worked crossword puzzles and even took out our old Scrabble game and tried to play by myself. Realizing how difficult this was unsettled me, but I persevered. Gradually, I improved. The halting speech occurred less frequently, but when I was tired, the same communication glitch surfaced, as if my brain were saying, "Sorry, gone on vacation!" This was indeed my body's way of reminding me that I was dealing with a damaged engine.

The bicycle accident had damaged both hemispheres of my brain. The damage was widespread, including a concussion in the right front temple area resulting in prefrontal lobe lesions and temporal lobe and motor cortex damage to the left hemisphere. My speech impairment, known as aphasia, resulted from the left hemisphere damage. People with this type of injury occasionally recover the ability to speak a foreign language, at least to some extent. This has not been the case for me. Any French words I now know I have had to relearn since my accident, and they are limited to common phrases frequently used in English.

Of great interest to me has been the change in the way I construct language—sentence and paragraph structure and their delivery. I learned to speak fluently when I was very young, and I could read and write before I started school. Before the accident, I remembered vividly events that occurred when I was still a toddler, in a few cases as young as eighteen months old. I never considered this good memory a remarkable trait. But I feel the loss of these language skills deeply.

I almost never used inappropriate grammar in my former life. After the accident, I had difficulty forming even the simplest sentence in the proper grammatical order. Eager to take part in a conversation, I sometimes responded by restating a question without readjusting the order of the subject and the verb. (My answer to "What colors do you like best?" might be "Blue colors do I like best.") The condition, known as "transcortical motor aphasia," resulted from damage to the temporal lobe and the motor cortex. It made it difficult for me to create new sentences or phrases and led to my halting speech.

After the accident, my speech patterns resembled those of Northern Europeans (Swedes, Norwegians, Germans) who learn English as a second language. They tend to translate their words into English literally while retaining the Northern European structure, which places the action verb at the end of the sentence. Interestingly, my great-grandparents, who lived nearby, spoke these languages around me when I was a child.

I found the limerick below in *A Treasury of Children's Poetry*. It reminded me of the need to maintain a sense of humor while dealing with the hard work of recovery. I usually kept samples of silly, light reading near my favorite chair. Children's whimsical poems proved to be a delight as did stories of pets. I particularly related to this poem.

## I Left My Head
by Lillian Moore (American writer, 1909–2004)

I left my head somewhere today,
Put it down for just a minute.
Under the table? On a chair?
Wish I were able to say where.
Everything I need is in it!

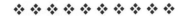

*In Retrospect:*

I found it hard to determine whether the brain damage or the hearing deficiency led to my impaired language skills. In many ways it did not matter, because in the early stages I simply worked as steadily as I could to regain as many of my lost skills as possible. Dr. Joseph Corbett had warned me that my cognitive skills might be impaired, so I set out to reread books I had read years ago, starting with simple text. At first I could read for only half an hour before the effort exhausted me. I exercised in this way every day, gradually increasing the time spent in reading and in writing, with the requisite dictionary and thesaurus nearby.

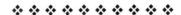

*Medical Descriptions:*

Damage done to my frontal lobe was complex. This area of the brain controls several language functions, among them expressive language, understanding the meaning of words, and word associations. The damage to the left temporal lobe, in addition to affecting my hearing, caused problems related to language such as difficulty in understanding spoken words and difficulty identifying objects and naming them. I experienced all of these problems to varying degrees.

*Medical Definitions:*

aphasia—impairment or loss of faculty using or understanding
    spoken or written language.

# 8

# Executive in the Kitchen

"I DID IT!" I said triumphantly to my cat, Shadow, as we settled into the Boston rocker in the lower den. With much care and calculation, I had made a delicious cup of coffee—a real accomplishment now—and toasted an English muffin, which I had spread with butter and my homemade strawberry jam. Now I was enjoying my treat.

I never had owned an automatic coffee maker and used to scoff at the thought of purchasing one. Although buying a coffee maker made sense now, I resolved to master the skill of making a cup of coffee again. That morning, a little more than a month after my accident, I boiled water, measured coffee beans, and then ground them. I filled a filter-lined cone with the ground coffee. The cone balanced on my thermal carafe, and I calculated how much boiling water to pour into the opening so as not to overfill the container. This process had always produced a nice cup of kaffe—true to my Scandinavian roots—appropriately rich but not acidic. Now once again I was able to accomplish the task. Shadow purred in appreciation. I felt like purring myself.

The jam came from one of the few remaining jars from last year's preserving. I sipped the hot coffee and nibbled on the muffin, savoring each bite. I wondered if I would ever be able to make jam again.

After the accident, preparing the simplest of meals became incredibly complex for me. I agonized over each step:

1.  purchase ingredients,
2.  prepare tools,
3.  mix ingredients in proper order, and finally,
4.  schedule preparation so that all dishes are ready to be served together.

For years I had carelessly taken the ability to cook for granted. Now I developed a deep appreciation for the skills it took to create a simple meal. Nearly every area of my damaged brain came into play as I struggled to accomplish the mundane act of preparing even a sandwich and a cup of coffee. Short-term and long-term memory problems surfaced; I no longer could rely on a keen sense of taste and smell; I had difficulty doing things in the proper order. The clinical term for these abilities is executive skills, and I needed every one of them to learn to cook again.

To recover my taste and smell, I began nibbling crystallized ginger, reputed to expand membranes in the sinus region. (And nibble was all I could do with that powerful spice.) One sense affects the other; my limited sense of taste decreased my ability to smell. The corda tympani nerve of the middle ear transmits taste to both sides of the tongue. The damage done to my left ear affected my total response even though the nerve on my right side remained intact. All of this affected my ability to taste spices, sample recipes, and perform other necessary tasks essential in cooking.

After we had eaten the food our friends had provided, I

wondered how we would cope with everyday food preparation? I could not understand my recipes, and Ted was hopeless when it came to cooking. His solution was always to visit the corner diner. I did not always want to eat out; sometimes I wanted to dine at home and eat home-cooked food. And I wanted to be able to cook again.

A note from my journal, September 22, 1990:

*A Prayer to be said when "'the world has gotten you down, and you feel rotten, and you're too doggone tired to pray, and you're in a big hurry, and besides, you're mad at everybody— HELP!" I don't know why asking for help is so hard. It's actually smart. It's the answer to fatigue and the "I'm indispensable" image. But something keeps me from this smart move, maybe something as simple as pride. I fear the greatest battle I may face is not inefficiency but super-efficiency, the person who never lets anyone down, the person who is ALWAYS TRYING TO HOLD IT ALL TOGETHER—AND DOES! Question, "Will I ever be super-efficient again?"*

On September 23, 1990, a Sunday afternoon, Adam and his friend Dave came downstairs and headed for the cookie jar. Grabbing a handful of Oreos and a quart of milk, they headed outside to throw a ball. Adam said, "Hey, Mom, when are you going to make some more of your famous chocolate chip cookies? I sure do miss them. It's been a while."

"Yea," Dave added with a grin. "Football players need to keep their strength up."

I smiled. "How's your mom, Dave?"

"She's fine. Said for me to tell you she said 'Hi.' She's in between jobs right now, but she's doing okay."

"Hey, Mom, maybe we should get Shirley to come down

and help you out," Adam said in a whisper and gave my back a quick stroke. "We'll be outside." Then, raising his voice a bit, he called, "Hey, Demers, I'm ready to beat you!" And with that the two boys dashed outside.

What a good idea! I immediately went in search of Ted. Before the week was up, we had hired my friend Shirley Demers, who was a nurse's aide, to help me regain my health and perform the many household chores that needed to be done. She came several days a week and cooked, cleaned, swept the floors, and washed the clothes. Her biggest contribution was her boundless patience as she helped me cope with my own discouragement and encouraged me to relearn simple tasks. With humor and common sense, we implemented Dr. Shedd's directives and added a few ideas of our own. It was a comfort to have Shirley around.

Shirley became my guide as I faced my fears and slowly overcame them. We knew we had succeeded when we could laugh about the ordeal afterward. Going down stairs continued to be a real challenge. My balance was so impaired that I had a great fear of falling forward. Shirley walked down ahead of me, and I steadied myself with my hand on her shoulder as we descended together.

In the kitchen, she became provider and teacher. She prepared extra entrees for us to eat on the days she was not with us, but she also taught me to prepare simple meals using my own recipe books. Her greatest gift was my sense of accomplishment and independence after I mastered a favorite recipe.

"Let's start with some chocolate chip cookies for Adam," she said on one of her first days with us. Class had begun. My recipe book opened to a well-stained page with handwritten notes of how I had adapted old, familiar recipes. Shirley smiled.

"Looks like your handwriting, Kitty."

I had to agree. The writing was definitely mine. Tears welled up as I tried to figure out the procedure that had once been so easy. Shirley patted my hand.

"We'll do this together. First we need a big bowl and measuring cups and spoons. Remember the baking sheet."

I took a deep breath and pulled out the kitchen tools.

"You crossed out 'one package brown sugar' and wrote in 'one cup granulated sugar and one cup dark brown sugar.' And you replaced 'one cup shortening' with '½ cup soft butter and ½ cup shortening.' So first we take out these items: dark brown sugar, white sugar, butter, and shortening. We'll measure these out and dump them in the bowl." Shirley spoke calmly and confidently, with a smile on her face. "Let's wash our hands first."

After we had washed our hands, she asked me to read the rest of the ingredients in the recipe.

"Two unbeaten eggs and one teaspoon vanilla," I read aloud. "It says to beat these together with the sugar and shortening."

"Okay, let's get out the electric beater. Will it bother you to use this?" she asked.

"I don't know," I said as I pulled out the electric beater. "We can try."

Shirley showed me how to insert the beaters into the appropriate holes and cautioned me not to plug in the mixer until after I had checked to make sure the beaters were secure. The beater vibrated as I held it in the batter. I felt shaky but completed the task. Shirley reached for the mixer. First stage done. I drew a deep breath and smiled. Shirley smiled back and patted my shoulder.

"Now we have to preheat the oven," Shirley said. "Read the recipe, Kitty. What temperature does it ask for?" She pointed to the page and directed my eyes to the temperature reading.

"It says 350 degrees for ten to fifteen minutes, but I crossed out the fifteen, so I must have baked them for only ten minutes," I told her.

"Apparently your boys like a soft cookie, so you baked them for less time. The longer they are in the oven, the drier they become," Shirley explained. "Turn the oven to 350 to warm up as we finish preparing the batter," Shirley instructed. "What more does the recipe call for?"

"Three cups sifted flour, one teaspoon soda, two teaspoons cream of tartar, salt—this doesn't say how much, Shirley. What do I do?" Shirley looked over my shoulder, reaching for another bowl along with a sifter.

"That's okay. When it doesn't say, it just means a shake or two. Let's measure out these dry ingredients into this big bowl. We'll use the sifter to mix it all together as we measure." We set the sifter into the big bowl and measured the flour and other ingredients into it. The two bowls, one with the dry mixture and the other with the buttery egg mixture sat in front of us on the counter.

"Now we combine the two bowls. We can either use the electric mixer, our clean hands, or a big spoon and a lot of muscle. Which one do you want to use, Kitty?" I saw the twinkle in her eye as she started to remove rings from her fingers. She knew hands would be my preferred tool. So our rings came off, and we kneaded the dry ingredients into the moist ones. Then came the chocolate chips, added last.

When we had thoroughly mixed the batter, we left it and washed our hands and cleaned the work surface. Spooning batter into balls onto the baking sheet, we fashioned several dozen cookies. Afterward, as we treated ourselves to a cup of tea and a delicious, homemade cookie. I felt triumphant and so thankful for Shirley's help.

"Does any of what we did seem familiar?" she asked.

"Yes and no," I replied. "I remember making cookies, but I don't recall the specifics of how I did it. But at least my own recipe books don't seem quite like the maze they did before."

"What's with the electric beater? It bothered you, didn't it? Was it the noise?" Curiosity mixed with concern in her voice.

"Mostly it was the vibration," I said. "It made me dizzy. That's odd, isn't it?"

Shirley just smiled, patted my hand, and said, "We'll make a note to tell your doctor about it. Next time we'll tackle the pot roast. No electric beaters with that one!"

"Sounds good," I said and meant it.

In this slow and methodical way, we worked through the cookbooks. I relearned the meaning of preparation terms: braise, sear, broil, and so on. What a relief to be able to cook my own food! I was encouraged by my progress, even if I still needed a guide in the kitchen. Shirley did not mind that I could not remember some words and needed to write down every instruction, then check it off as we completed the task. Her compassion was boundless, her humor at the ready. Since I was surrounded by men in my life, it was a relief to talk to a woman for a change.

It is unfortunate that we often overlook the obvious. No one expects someone with a broken leg to get up and dance. But after my body healed on the outside, it was easy for Ted, Guy, and Adam to presume I was equally healed on the inside. I was not. I did not discuss my brokenness; neither did the rest of the family. Such a discussion would have revealed my continuing need for help and encouragement. But those conversations never took place.

That Thanksgiving proved to be one of the most discouraging times of my recovery. I knew I would not be able to handle all the complex tasks involved in preparing our holiday meal, as I always had in the past. Guy and Adam planned to spend the day with us, but Ted's youngest daughter, Teri, would be with her mother. The older girls would celebrate with their boyfriends' families.

To prepare for the holiday, Shirley baked pies, and she and I bought rolls, vegetables, and a pre-stuffed turkey. I hoped Guy and Adam could prepare a simple holiday meal if I gathered all the necessary ingredients ahead of time. When I presented the plan for Thanksgiving to them, they were thunderstruck that I could not, or, in their minds, would not, prepare the meal.

On the big day I set the table, then had to rest. Ted retreated to the safety of his study and his computer, muttering as he went that he "should have made a reservation at a restaurant." In the kitchen Guy and Adam quietly grumbled as they tried to figure out how to cook a turkey, peel potatoes, and prepare carrots, squash, and peas.

"Don't forget the cranberry sauce," I heard Adam say.

"Do we really need gravy?" asked Guy. "What's stuffed celery? We can just put celery on a plate, can't we?"

"Oh, sure," Adam replied. "Mom won't care. She said we can do what we want, just cook the bird and vegetables."

We ate Thanksgiving dinner a bit later than planned, but we got through it all. Ted, having mastered the dishwasher, cleaned up after the meal. No one mentioned the "elephant in the room," my failure to fill my traditional role as cook and chief bottle-washer. That topic remained buried as did the feelings surrounding it. We did not discuss the resentment of the boys and Ted that I was not resuming my kitchen duties now that my wounds had healed. I did not talk about my disability and my needs or my feeling that I was letting them all down.

When Shirley came the next day, we had a long chat. She

provided needed ballast when things became stormy. Sometimes girlfriends are a lifeline.

*In Retrospect:*

An occupational therapist and a family counselor could have provided us with valuable services that would have made my recovery much easier. They might have been able to help each family member know what to expect from me and what I needed from them. This would have strengthened the family. Unfortunately, we did not utilize those services.

Family counseling might have revealed that Ted had several challenges of his own that limited how he could help. Counseling sessions might also have shown that Guy and Adam, involved in their own young lives, had adopted a hands-off attitude toward their divorced parents' problems. Their dad and I had many unresolved feelings after our divorce and that made it difficult for the boys to become overly involved in either parent's life.

I was unaccustomed to asking for help and had never been good at voicing my needs. It never occurred to me, or anyone else, to change the ways we all related to one another within the family to ease my difficult healing journey. Looking back, I regret not holding a family caucus; but in the midst of the day-to-day work I had to do to recover, I did not have the objectivity or the astuteness to do so.

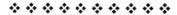

*Medical Description:*

Functions controlled by the frontal lobe of the cerebral cortex are involved in several areas of activities:

1.  consciousness within an environment,

2. initiation of activity,
3. daily judgments,
4. emotional response,
5. expressive language,
6. word association and ascribing meaning to the words we use, and
7. memory of habits and motor activities.

Frontal lobe damage primarily affects day-to-day activities and can result in:

1. an inability to plan a sequence of complex movements needed to complete multistepped tasks, such as making coffee. (This is normally referred to as sequencing.)
2. a loss of flexibility in thinking.
3. an inability to focus on a task (attending).
4. the persistence of a single thought (perseveration).
5. a difficulty with problem solving.
6. the inability to express language (aphasia).

Many of these functions are combined under the title "executive function." The executive function controls the ability to organize, plan, and follow through in the abstract.

\* \* \* \* \*

Almost a year after Shirley began teaching me to cook again, I noted real success in my journal. From my journal, September 4, 1991:

> *I am so pleased with myself that when dear friends Irene and Barbara were here visiting from Florida, we were able to host them in a "normal fashion" and with seeming ease. I was actually able to pull together an impromptu light meal of homemade tomato bisque*

*soup! Yea! It was a small thing to be sure, but so very WONDERFUL to be able to do. It was SO VERY GOOD TO SEE THEM AND HAVE A WONDERFUL VISIT!! Thank You, Lord. Wait 'til I tell Shirley and Judy [Dr. Shedd]. They will be pleased for me.*

Longtime friends Barbara Leslie and Irene Lee arrived from Florida in early September 1991. I had not seen them since before the accident. They arrived in the early afternoon. We were thrilled to have a chance to visit. Ted had told them of my accident, and they had kept me daily in their prayers.

We spoke often on the phone, but this was their first opportunity to see me face-to-face. Barbara was a nurse and no doubt had cautioned Irene not to step in and do things for me that I needed to do for myself. They both had experience with other friends who had recovered from strokes, so they were sensitive to the need for the recovering patient to set her own pace.

Irene particularly enjoyed Ted. He regaled her with stories that always produced laughter. We enjoyed one another's company and didn't want to interrupt the warm camaraderie by going to the diner for a meal. I went to the kitchen and decided to make tomato bisque with cheddar cheese slices and crackers. It was my great-grandmother's recipe.

Barbara came with me to the kitchen and sat on a stool as we chatted and I worked. She was careful not to distract me. I slowly melted three tablespoons of butter in a large saucepan. Carefully following the directions, I sliced a medium onion and added it to the butter, sautéing it until the mixture was shiny. In another pan I measured three tablespoons of cornstarch, added one cup of milk, and stirred until the mixture was smooth. I added the milk mixture to the onions and butter and stirred with a fork until the liquid thickened.

Only a few more steps to the finish. I added salt, pepper, more milk, and a large can of diced tomatoes. I kept the burner at medium low, heating the soup through. After a tentative taste, I added about a teaspoon of sugar to offset the acidity of the tomatoes. Done! I beamed with delight over my first triumph in the kitchen without help. Barbara smiled back at me and set the table.

Years before, I remembered visiting a dear missionary friend, Alma, who was recovering from a stroke. Alma preferred to handle her own recovery at her log cabin on a lake. As a person with severe diabetes, Alma had learned to be highly disciplined in taking care of her body as she continued to work vigorously for the cause she believed in. She had lived alone for many years after losing both her husband and her only child. Coming back to the lakeside cabin to heal was right for her. Barbara, Irene, and others tried to help Alma as much as possible, but all respected her solitary status and knew she had to find her own way.

In June 1982 I found myself practically sitting on my hands in Alma's kitchen as she methodically cut carrots to boil for our lunch. Potatoes were already cooking. I had brought ground beef to contribute to the meal. As I visited with Alma in that warm kitchen, I knew she needed to be able to prepare the meal for us more than I needed a meal. It would certainly have gone much faster if I had taken over her kitchen that day. But it would not have been a gift to her. My gift to her was to let her do the work.

Almost ten years later, as Barbara sat in my kitchen, practically sitting on her hands, I knew she was giving me a gift, and I was very grateful.

# 9

# On the Road Again

IN THE SPRING OF 1991 Ted and I realized that Teri, now eleven, no longer enjoyed riding her bicycle. Although she had a helmet and a safe bike and had been a good rider, she was hesitant and reluctant to go bicycling. Her fears appeared to be directly related to my accident. I knew the only way to get Teri past her fears would be to let her see me confront my own.

I worked hard to regain my sense of balance. By August 1991 I thought I had made enough progress to mount a bike again. I had not used a cane for several months and considered myself generally steady.

On the day of the trial run, Ted swallowed his own butterflies, fetched the helmets, and checked all the equipment to be sure it was in proper working order.

We involved Teri in the project. Her job was to roller-blade next to me in case I needed help. Fortunately, she took her assignment seriously. I'm not sure I could have done it without her.

My mind may have been ready for the challenge, but my body pushed for a delay. I perched on the bicycle seat and put one foot on the pedal. But when I went to lift the other foot, it remained glued to the ground. It seemed my foot had a mind of its own! For a time it refused to leave the safety of the ground to operate the other pedal.

"Come on, Kitty," Teri coaxed. "You can do it."

I took a deep breath, looked at Teri, and received her encouraging smile. That girl was so beautiful, I could not let her down. I could not allow her to fear riding her bike because of my accident.

I silently counted to ten, gave Teri a quick wink, then said, "Let's go."

And Teri cheered. She had a huge grin on her face as she proudly guided me along the roadway that circled our cul-de-sac. The day was clear and sunny, but I hardly noticed in my effort to concentrate on staying steady on the bike.

Teri glided along beside me, coaching me as we rounded the curves. "You're doing great, Kitty. Not much farther now. Hold steady as we slow down. Remember the bike tips some as you brake."

I turned into our driveway and pulled to a stop. Beaming, Teri circled around to face me. Her hands went up to signal a winning goal. As I safely dismounted, I saw Ted finally exhale a big sigh, as if he had held his breath during the entire ride.

We had hot fudge sundaes afterward to celebrate. I did not ride far. But I did ride successfully. And Teri rode her bike with much more confidence after that.

# 10

# Arts, Crafts, and Creativity

DURING MY FINAL EXAMINATION with Dr. Joseph Corbett, the neurosurgeon warned me that I should expect a serious loss of creativity. That upset me a great deal.

Creativity had always been a big part of who I was as a person. I enjoyed making my own patterns, painting, drawing, and combining subtle colors to create pleasing designs. Losing my ability to be creative would be a serious loss indeed. The doctor's warning scared me, and I prayed he was wrong.

As the months went on and I struggled with even mundane tasks, I realized that, as Dr. Corbett had predicted, the creative me had disappeared. Whether the loss would be permanent or temporary, I did not know. Nevertheless, I decided to focus on regaining simple skills in the hopes that my successes would ultimately spark my creative flow.

During the winter of 1990 and 1991, Ted and I read all we could find on the brain and creativity. I hoped that the research would teach me ways to stimulate my lost creativity. I found little that was helpful. Most of the studies used men in their research tests. Reading the results, I wondered if women might use different approaches.

One article* of interest focused on the correlation between lyrical sounds and art. The findings, from an art and music teacher who studied youngsters with advanced development in art, revealed that the Asian children in the study had superior fine-motor skills than American children of the same age. When the Asian youngsters were compared with American youngsters who came from musical households, the differences were not as significant. Brain wave tests showed that the same area that is stimulated by music is also stimulated by the sounds of the tonal Asian language. The article concluded that musical sounds may stimulate creative ability and fine-motor development.

The research confirmed my observations when I had taught art to children during a stint as substitute teacher years earlier. The Cambodian children in my class seemed to be more creative in their use of color and their manipulation of complicated forms than the other students. The younger Asian children also seemed more dexterous than their classmates.

Would listening to music at home help me? We searched through our collection of compact discs for music that was soothing and easy to listen to. Thereafter, we often had classical instrumentals playing in the background.

Another encouraging report came by way of conversations with a visiting professor of psychology, Laura Sewall. That winter Ted and I attended a series of lectures open to the public and held at the nearby University of New England. When I told Dr. Sewall of my accident, she urged me to continue in my rehabilitation efforts. She cited recent test studies on brain-damaged monkeys who had become fully functioning by making use of

---

*Vincent, Marilyn C. and Margaret Merrion. "The Musical Mind Considered: A New Frontier." *Design for Arts in Education.* Sept/Oct. 1990: 11–18.

parts of their brains that had not been used before. This news encouraged me to persevere. Two phrases—"keep on keeping on" and "listen to good music" became my mantras and gave me a sense of hope.

In spring 1991 Ted and I attended a conference for lumber manufacturers. As part-owner of a lumber concern, Ted had been a past president of the group and wanted to stay in touch with the other members. While he listened to lectures, I attended a program for the spouses on how to make floral wreaths. I sat in the front row where I could hear and see well. The instructor had put all the necessary items for wreath making on the work tables in front of us. I concentrated on the demonstration, trying to follow the instructions. Although the wreath I made differed slightly from the others on the table, it looked fine. But I could not seem to make a bow. Finally, the instructor came to look at my work.

"It's lovely," she said. "But since you're left-handed, let me show you another approach for the bow that will work better." She reached across the workbench for a pink ribbon.

"But I'm right-handed," I protested.

The instructor was adamant. "The flow of this wreath definitely has a left-handed approach. Beautiful, but clearly left-handed. Now let's try this bow."

A bit shocked since I had always considered myself right-handed, I followed orders and completed the bow, using my right hand but following the much-easier left-handed directions. When I finished, I admired my handiwork, but I rejoiced even more in the revelation it had brought. My newfound left-handedness gave me hope that new connections had begun to form in my brain.

Encouraged by my few attempts at crafts, I decided to try to relearn the skills involved in the creative activities I had once pursued. I began with knitting. I did not dare finish any knitted project started before my accident. The difference in skill level would have been too noticeable. My first attempts at knitting simple sampler swatches turned out to be incredibly difficult.

Fortunately, my fundamental skill books provided diagrams for both right-handed and left-handed learners. Although I still considered myself right-handed, I could make no sense of the written instructions for right-handed knitters. Only as I looked at diagrams for left-handed people did the instructions become clear. I continued to use my right hand but followed the instructions for left-handed knitters on the diagram.

Learning to knit and crochet again was akin to learning a challenging foreign language. I had to concentrate on every stitch as if each were a word that needed to be translated. This was true even when the stitch was a repeat of the previous stitch. For each project, I studied the diagram, pulled the yarn over the tip of the needle while holding it firm, and then guided the needle and pulled the yarn through. That stitch completed, I had to look again at the diagram to place the needles and the yarn in the proper position for the next stitch—which was a repeat of the last one. I took no joy in doing this tedious work; I settled for relief and quiet triumph. Joy would come later.

I had begun to knit cotton dish clothes, which I determinedly produced in a variety of colors. After I had knitted one for everyone I knew, I graduated to a few other small items. The insightful comment of a dear man, my husband's elder cousin, encouraged me to try more challenging projects. Before my accident I had started to knit a Nordic vest for my father. I had set it aside in the summer months, not wanting to work with wool in the heat. Then I had the accident, and for a year I was afraid to work on the vest again.

A breakthrough came when Ted and I visited Don and Ellie

Saunders in early fall 1991. We settled around the coffee table in the front sitting room of their old colonial. Ellie brought in a tray of tea and cookies. They were a gracious couple, beautifully suited to each other, it seemed. Free of other distracting sounds, we concentrated on each other in this soothing environment. My recovery process came up in conversation.

Gently, but pointedly, Don asked, "So, Kitty, what, in all of this, are you most afraid of?"

"Creativity," I answered without hesitation. "I'm most frightened that I might not be able to reclaim my creativity in fine-motor skills like knitting, crocheting, embroidery, and painting. These were always important ways of expressing myself. One of my doctors warned me, though, that my creativity may be lost forever." Don listened quietly, sensing that I was mourning a treasured part of myself that had died, or so I had been told.

"I am trying to learn to knit again," I confided. "It is very challenging. It takes me forever to do just a very small thing. I have a Nordic vest that I had started for my father before the accident, but I'm afraid to try to finish it because I think the stitches will be very different now. My dad may never get his vest."

Don put his fingertips together and looked at me with his penetrating gaze. "Kitty, I know your father. And I do believe he will value the vest more from you now, complete with different stitches, than he ever would have before."

And I knew he was right. As soon as Ted and I got home, I dug out the unfinished vest and called my friend, Betty Ann Hammond, the owner of a knitting shop. I made an appointment to take lessons.

Dad received his vest the following May on his seventy-sixth birthday. Pulling the gray and cream-colored wool vest out of the package, he looked at me and smiled broadly. The sweater featured a gray deer I had replicated in wool from the design on the vest's pewter buttons. Nordic snowflakes lined the border. "This is real nice. You've done a fine job." He proudly put it on. His voice had the same touch of pride when he told admirers of the sweater that his daughter Kitty had made it for him.

After that I learned to sew clothes and quilts again. Reading patterns for left-handed crafters and implementing them with my right hand remains a challenge. But it is worth the effort to be able to create things that bring pleasure to me and to loved ones who receive them as gifts.

In the summer of 1991 a small notice in the newspaper caught my eye. It advertised a one-afternoon session of "Turning Memories into Memoirs" with writer Denis Ledoux. I signed up for the class. The session inspired me to record anecdotes from my childhood as a way of telling my story to my children. I had three thoughts in mind: I wanted my family to know me and understand the significant people and events that had shaped me, I wanted to reexamine my family's history for myself, and I knew that the accounts of the challenges endured by my immigrant ancestors would help put my problems in perspective and give me added courage.

I knew I could not accomplish this alone, so in August 1991 I joined a writers group that had recently formed. We met monthly at the local library in Saco to read our work aloud and hear constructive comments from other writers. These monthly writing exercises proved invaluable in my endeavors to express myself and discipline my mind to produce clear thoughts. They also served to strengthen my self-identity and my self-esteem. Hearing what others had written also made me realize I was not alone in my struggles with expression. We shared a common goal; our particular paths might be different, but the challenges were the same.

## The Big Work

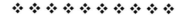

*In Retrospect:*

A friend had a plaque on her desk to remind herself of her value as a person. It said, "I am a human-being, not a human-doing!" With consistent work, I was becoming more capable in some skills, yet a nagging question hung like a shroud over me: "What conditions are going to be permanent, and can I live with them?"

Before the accident, much of my life had been defined by activities and accomplishments. With the loss of many of the skills I had once possessed, I longed to become known, accepted, and loved as I was now, limitations and all. Would I still be accepted by people and by myself if I could no longer "do" what I had once done?

My writers group helped fill that need within me. My self-esteem began to blossom as I reexamined the lives of important family members who had influenced me. Dr. Roy P. Fairfield, original mentor of the writers group, nourished the belief that the individual creative spirit had authenticity and value. He taught me not to be frightened of speaking my mind. He invited me to come out of my shell and reveal myself as I was. He nurtured my creative flame and gave me hope.

The exercise of writing a story, reading it aloud, and listening as the class critiqued it proved to be therapeutic. This validating experience was a direct contrast to other parts of my life. Many people in my circle of friends and family could not seem to accept the extent of my injuries. In the face of this resistance, I rarely spoke of my limitations. Denial, even my own sense of denial, prevented all of us from growing and meeting the challenges demanded by my condition. As a result, communication within the family, in particular, lacked depth. We tended to avoid topics that dealt with real concerns and real feelings.

My struggle to recover basic skills left me exhausted, frightened, and sometimes very discouraged. The writing of family vignettes helped me reclaim a sense of who I was and led me to understand that I, too, was "a human-being, not just a human-doing."

*Medical Description:*

Damage to my frontal lobe, parietal lobe, and temporal lobe affected areas of my brain linked to creativity and artistic abilities. Among other things, the parietal lobe controls eye-and-hand coordination and the ability to distinguish left from right. The difficulties I encountered while learning how to knit, crochet, and sew again could be traced to the damaged temporal lobe, which caused similar problems in language skills. Temporal lobes regulate memory acquisition, visual perceptions, and categorization of objects.

# 11

# Visual Challenges

FROM MY JOURNAL, September 4, 1991:

*I'm still doing it, working diligently on a project, and Ted interrupts me by sliding a paper into my line of vision to ask me a question. I snap at him. I don't mean to be angry, but it hurts my head when he does this, and I don't know why! It isn't like he is hitting me—he's not, he is merely trying to get my attention in as polite a way as possible. Why does that hurt my head? I must talk to Judy [Dr. Shedd] about this. It makes no sense.*

With a family history of glaucoma and cataracts, I knew I should have my eyes tested at least every two years. We delayed my regular eye appointment while waiting for my cranial swelling to subside. Since I had not reported any new vision problems, we had not rushed to reschedule the appointment. Headaches had been an ongoing problem for me, but we assumed they were related to the accident, not a visual problem. I had worn tinted glasses to improve my long-distance vision while driving for years. In fall 1991, Dr. Shedd suggested I see an eye doctor with experience in head injury cases.

On December 6, 1991, my father drove me to Concord, New Hampshire, for my first appointment with Dr. James Mancini, an optometrist who had treated many patients with head injuries. Through a series of questions as well as the examination, the doctor determined that the muscles around my eyes had been damaged, resulting in an eye problem known as convergence excess. The condition caused my eyes to lock in place when I focused on an object. This severely restricted my field of vision, resulting in a form of tunnel vision that forced me to focus on only one object at a time.

After the accident, I found it difficult to switch tasks or to focus on more than one task at a time. My response reminded me of an old-fashioned train that had to stop and wait until a switch could be pulled before it could proceed onto a new set of tracks.

When Ted asked me a question not related to the work at hand, I could not reply. I became impatient with him if he interrupted my train of thought. To avoid disturbing me, he wrote messages on pieces of paper and slipped them gently within my line of vision when he needed to get my attention. Not only did the action interrupt my thoughts; it also hurt me physically, causing a sharp pain in my head. I crossly told Ted not to repeat his actions, but he continued because he could not figure out how else to gain my attention.

Because of my eye condition, shifting to look at another object after my eyes locked into position caused pain. The condition also led me to focus with such intensity on a project that I forgot to take breaks, even to eat. After the consultation with Dr. Mancini, I installed a series of small clocks around the house. As I began a project, I looked at the clock and noted the time. I made it a point to work no more than an hour on a problem without taking a break. The clocks reminded me of that pledge and kept me on track. Dr. Mancini prescribed a series of visual exercises for me to follow. One involved a bead on a string, which I attached to a window ledge. As I moved the bead along the string, I learned to focus on it at different points. I did this several times a day for many months until the muscles around my eyes relaxed. The doctor also prescribed special glasses to correct the condition. Gradually, I improved. As I did, my ability to multitask began to improve as well.

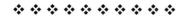

*In Retrospect:*

It is rather odd to realize that we solve problems based on how we see them. This becomes the literal truth for people with head injuries. I discovered that I could not handle a multitask problem because my vision could focus on only one thing at a time. Once my vision problem was addressed, I was able to shift my attention (as well as my sight) from one thing to another more easily.

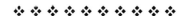

*Medical Description:*

The brain controls visual functions, among them the way one object is perceived to relate to another (spatial perception). Damage to the frontal lobe and the parietal lobe as well as the occipital lobes all contributed to my visual problems. The frontal lobe damage affected my ability to plan a sequence of complex movements needed to complete multistepped tasks; it also caused me to remain focused on a single thought. The damage to the parietal lobe made it difficult for me to draw and to apply mathematics. It also interfered with my ability to multitask. The occipital lobes damage impaired my reading and writing skills and prevented me from focusing on more than one object at a time within my range of vision. Fortunately, I did not experience other problems that have been associated with damage to the occipital lobes, such as difficulty in distinguishing colors, total or moderate blindness, and hallucinations.

## Anniversary

It was a ride I'll never forget,
Yet can never remember—
    The intended bike ride,
    Then waking up six days later
    In a pale green hospital room
Set on a path of rebuilding,
    Reparenting   Relearning
        Reconnecting,
Forging new connections
Within the broken parts of me.
It had been one thing
        To teach the handicapped.
It was something else
        To become handicapped.
And yet, with so much taken away,
I've not plumbed the depth
    Of me
        And my ability to grow.
I know
        We were created
    With incredible possibilities.
We can
        Become amazing beings,
  If we choose.

EAC/1992

# Section III

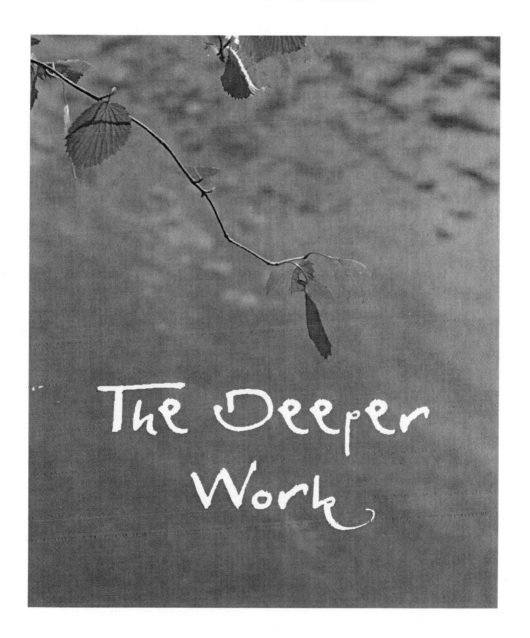

The Deeper Work

# Sandpaper

I've met veneered people,
but I cannot join
their society.
I am called
to a very plain society—
where I am the same
inside as outside—
just me—
just as I am.
I know this because
I have been surrounded
by sandpaper people,
who would simply ruin
good veneer.

EAC/1993

# 12

# Attitude Is Everything

PEOPLE HAVE ASKED ME if I was ever depressed. The answer is yes, many times. On Thursday, September, 13, 1990, I had been home less than three weeks, and the pain seemed endless. The fear that it would never end hung over me like a shroud. I questioned God and heard no answer. I could not escape the uncertainty of my future. Would my life ever have any value to society if I could not achieve even simple things? When I left the hospital, I told the nurse I was not afraid, but as each day wore on, I found it increasingly more difficult to maintain that attitude. The old nursery rhyme kept interrupting my thoughts:

> Humpty Dumpty sat on a wall
> Humpty Dumpty had a great fall.
> All the king's horses and all the king's men
> Couldn't put Humpty together again.

It was easy to forget Dr. Judy Shedd's assurances that I would one day heal. Most of the time I felt like the broken Humpty Dumpty in the rhyme or was consumed by pain and confusion. After I had finally succeeded in tying my shoes on the fifth attempt, tears rolled down my face as I questioned what my future held. Simply moving was both painful and dizzying. My neurosurgeon, Dr. Joseph Corbett, had offered no clear hope of recovery. Discouraged and depressed, I faced a real test of my faith.

From my journal, Thursday, September 13, 1990:

> *My brother's birthday tomorrow—must phone him, but don't want to scare him by sounding discouraged—he'd hear it in my voice—must deal with this pain first— Oh, Lord, I'm tired of hurting. God, are you there? Do you even care? Lord, I had always assured my boys that you loved us with an everlasting love, and that you cared what happened to us. Was I lying to my sons? Because you seem so very far away. Lord, you have been my anchor and strength as I dealt with many past troubles. Please don't abandon me now.*

I read Psalms, Proverbs, and Jeremiah from my Bible. Psalms 119:105—"Thy word is a lamp unto my feet, and a light unto my path"—spoke strongly to me. I remembered that in biblical times people walked with small lamps attached to their feet to light the pathway ahead. I certainly felt as if I were on an unlit path. I truly needed a lamp to light my way.

As I read the Bible verses, I realized if I did not proceed in blind faith on the path of recovery—whatever that recovery would be—my faith would appear false, a mere faith of convenience. I knew there was a real gap between my feelings and the faith I had professed for so long. I had certainly made mistakes in my life; no doubt people close to me could attest to that. I did not want to be a religious hypocrite. I did not believe that because I was a Christian, I should be exempt from trauma and pain. The Bible is filled with examples of good Jews and Christians who suffered terrible problems.

I had been given life when I easily could have died. Although I was discouraged and afraid, suicide was not an option. I had lived through my mother's suicide years before. Intellectually I understood her choice in light of the health problems that plagued her; emotionally I almost drowned in the feeling of abandonment. I did not want my family ever to experience that as the result of my actions. We cannot choose the legacy we inherit, but we can determine the legacy we leave.

I opened my journal. Written at the top margin of that day's page was a quote from Henry Ward Beecher, "God asks no man whether he will accept life. That is not the choice. You must take it. The only choice is how." I sat there stunned.

If I believed that God held all my tomorrows, then I had to leave those tomorrows with God and deal with what had been handed to me, the present. How I faced my present challenges would be my legacy whether I was able to regain lost skills again or not. Perhaps my only legacy would be just showing up and cheering others on. It felt as if I had been led to an obscure path on a foggy night, without a map or a light, and told to step forward. Only in pure faith could I take that step and presume that I would find the earth beneath me.

I stepped forward.

Written in the margin near Psalm 119 I had made a notation to see Jeremiah 29:11–14. I turned there and read:

> For I know the thoughts that I think towards you,
> saith the Lord, thoughts of peace, and not of evil,
> to give you a future and a life.

I inhaled deeply, wiped my tears away, and quietly prayed, *Lord, if I survive this, don't let my future be one of just politely, dutifully standing by as others whisper and nod, saying, "Isn't it sad, she can't even tie her sneakers!"*

When I talked with Dr. Shedd at her office the next day, she reminded me that I had a body that wanted to heal. She assured me that step by step we would create an environment where healing could best take place. She told me to write my own prescription for wellness and read it to myself three times a day.

I wrote in my journal that day:

*1. God gave me a body that wants to be healthy.*

*2. Picture myself succeeding.*

*3. Dwell in the positive not the negative.*

*4. Give thanks daily.*

*5. Ask God to give me new dreams for each tomorrow.*

My father-in-law phoned a few days later to see how I was doing and asked if I was depressed. By then I could say, "No." I told him that I knew we could not control the problems that came our way, but we certainly could control the way we looked at those problems. I felt blessed. I had a lot to be thankful for.

It dawned on me that I had to commit anew to continued healing—whatever that healing would be. I was beginning to understand that recovering from brain injury is not like breaking an arm, wearing a cast, removing the cast, exercising the arm, then going back to pitching the softball. The legacy I would leave my loved ones might not be anywhere near what I had once hoped it would be; instead, it might only be a legacy of continuing to love family, commitment to my fellow man, and growing to the extent my brain could function. There might be many things I would never be able to do.

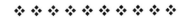

*In Retrospect:*

Years later I read Monique Le Poncin's *Brain Fitness,* an account of her clients' recuperation from traumatic brain injury. She observed that a person's return to "normal" is often quicker and more complete if he or she is strong-willed and has a resolute character. That was of primary importance in my case. I believe character is a manifestation of core values, and personality is how that character is expressed. My core values are rooted in a belief in *eternity,* which has always been a stabilizing force within me. From these core values came the perseverance required for my long journey of recovery.

# 13

# Anxieties and Fears

From my journal, Monday, November 5, 1990:

> *Realizing my balance was pretty bad, Dad came over
> yesterday with two canes he made for me—one was oak,
> the other was from an apple tree. He also brought a pair
> of deerskin loafers just my size. I'm grateful. Dad al-
> ways seems to anticipate what I am going to need next.
> Today I've resolved to sort through all my shoes. Shirley
> helped me. I cried a bit. I even tried to model a few of
> them before we both agreed they had to go. My balance
> was pathetic. We agreed that I surely would be a comic
> sight tottering unsteadily around in them. I particu-
> larly favored a pair of light blue high heels, but I put
> them in the bag like so many others. We took them to
> Goodwill. At least someone else could enjoy them. But
> these canes, they're beautiful because Dad made them,
> and he knows I need them—but, OH, I hope I don't
> need them for too long. It seems like another lifetime ago
> when I would dress up in pretty clothes and stylish high
> heels and dance. Will I ever do it again?*

Balance remained a challenge for a long time. I began using many of the tips provided by Dr. John Knowles, my ear specialist, to cope with the lack of balance. I knew I had to learn to walk again in a very different way.

Ted found some nearby hiking trails along the Saco River. We started hiking these wooded trails whenever the weather allowed. To prepare for tramping along the trails, I walked with Ted around our neighborhood cul-de-sac. My first attempts were uncertain and difficult. I walked slowly and unsteadily. Walking beside me on our first foray, Ted swept his foot across the path to clear it of pebbles and other impediments. That act, which he meant to be helpful, actually made me dizzier because of the effect on my brain of the image of his foot flashing in front of me. I cried out in alarm and almost fell. Startled, Ted steadied me. Once he understood the problem, he took care not to make sudden movements in front of me.

I tired easily, and my fear of falling haunted every step. Gradually I improved, but for some time I battled nausea whenever I walked on uneven ground. It took so little to throw me off balance.

From my journal, March 1, 1991:

> *My goal is to be able to walk with reasonable confidence through the field to the football stadium when Guy graduates this year. I'm doing fairly well coming down stairs now, thanks to Shirley, but uneven ground is still hard. And I know the crowds on graduation day will be overwhelming. I don't want to be a distraction from His Day. I'll mention this to Judy [Dr. Shedd]; perhaps she has some exercises to help me with balance.*

Dr. Judy Shedd arranged for me to meet with Carla Keene, a specialist in Trager therapy. Though Trager therapy feels like a thoroughly relaxing, gentle massage, it combines relaxation therapy and mental imaging designed to reeducate the body and make it receptive to healing and rejuvenation. Ms. Keene also instructed me in exercises to improve my balance. One required me to roll large marbles around on a rug with the soles of my feet. This helped sensitize my feet, which in turn aided in developing good balance. That summer I walked barefoot on the sand of nearby beaches, a once-a-week exercise also suggested by the therapist. Following instructions, I stopped midway along my walk to meditate, visualizing my feet as sandbags that hugged the ground and kept me steady.

When Guy graduated from the University of Maine in May of 1991, I still walked with a cane, but I had become less dependent on it than before. We drove almost three hours to attend the graduation exercises, held on the football field of the Orono campus. Spectators sat on high-rise bleachers. Dad and Ted took charge of guiding me up to a seat between them. At the end of the ceremonies, we carefully made our way down the bleachers. As I negotiated the steps, I focused on the skills I had learned walking down the stairs with Shirley in front of me. In that way I kept panic from taking over my mind.

\* \* \* \* \*

Dr. Shedd provided me with an invaluable guide when she arranged for me to meet one of her patients six months after my accident. Linda turned out to be a beloved friend and a source of much-needed encouragement. Whenever I became confused or frightened, I called Linda, and she talked me through the latest crisis.

Ten years earlier Linda had experienced the same type of accident that I had endured. Her accident occurred in a small town in western Massachusetts. At that time, in that hospital, doctors automatically removed a portion of the brain when severe swelling followed a head injury. After Linda was released from the hospital, her fiancé left her. Her doctors told her to expect only limited recovery. In desperation, she moved to Maine and lived alone at her aunt's rustic cabin. She cut and carried wood for heat and dealt with other household challenges. Many of those closest to Linda, those who knew of her ordeal and her limitations, thought she would never survive. She proved them wrong.

More than anyone else, Linda knew the challenges I faced. She warned against overstimulation, both visual and audio, and reminded me that my brain was a damaged organ that needed time to heal. But it *would* heal, she was proof of that. When I asked if she believed she had fully recovered, she replied, "I'm back 110 percent." I questioned that. She acknowledged she might never be able to do certain activities again. But she pointed out that she had learned new ways of doing things and had become much wiser in her decisions. She valued life more. Since the accident, she believed, her life had become richer and fuller. By her example, Linda cheered me and gave me the courage to face my fears.

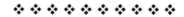

*In Retrospect:*

The support that comes from someone who has been there can be invaluable and in some cases life-saving. Recognizing this, TBI centers at rehabilitation clinics incorporate such support systems in their treatment of TBI patients. Many people can voice their fears and confusion only to someone who has been through the same challenges they face. Often they are more paralyzed by fear and confusion than by anything else during the recovery period.

When I began my rehabilitation, local TBI centers had not yet been established. A couple years after my accident Maine Medical Center, the Portland hospital where I received treatment, opened a TBI center. At that stage in my recovery, however, Dr. Shedd and I decided not to utilize the newly developing center. Since I was making good progress, Dr. Shedd feared that because I was by nature a compassionate person, I might spend more time trying to help others than focusing on helping myself. The TBI department at Maine Medical Center has become a well-established and respected center that does much good work. Likewise, the New England Rehabilitation Center, where Maine Medical Center sends its TBI patients for rehabilitation, has developed into a premier treatment facility for TBI.

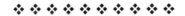

*Medical Description:*

I began Trager therapy in the late spring of 1991 to address balance problems and pain. I still experienced extreme pain on my left side, which was swollen and black and blue. To shrink the remaining hematomas on my left thigh, I applied vitamin E oil directly after hot showers and covered the area with a hot compress. The hematomas faded with this treatment, but the thigh remained swollen and painful. Several sessions of Trager therapy helped both conditions. Developed in the 1920s by Milton Trager, an American medical doctor, the treatment uses gentle massage to retrain the body to relax and return to its original healthy state. Often it is used to counteract rigidity caused from an assault to the body. After the session the patient learns "Mentastics" (mental gymnastics) to recreate the feeling of relaxation experienced during the treatment.

# 14

# Decisions, Decisions, Decisions

FROM MY JOURNAL, February 1, 1991:

> II Chronicles 23:19: "And he set the gatekeepers at the gates of the house of the Lord, so that no one who was in any way unclean should enter." Oh, Lord, I need a Gatekeeper—someone to filter all the stuff that comes at me with a ferocious constancy and I've lost my ability to sift. I receive a mailing with images of hurt puppies and I want to adopt them ALL. Of course I can't. It's not that what is coming to me is "clean" or "unclean," it's the difference between good, better, and best. It's the difference between compassion and an empathy that can become self-destructive. Lord, if ancient Israel needed a Gatekeeper for the temple, can't you give me a Gatekeeper now? In fact, I needed it YESTERDAY! Sorry, Lord, but I went to a lot of trouble to teach my boys critical thinking skills: now you need to teach me that, Father, because I've forgotten how and need to learn again. Show me how to parent myself.

When my new friend, Linda, warned me of the dangers of overstimulation, I knew immediately what she meant. Every sight and sound stimulated my brain. It seemed that everything emitted little shock waves that sent direct stimuli to a raw, exposed organ. I had no protective barrier to enable me to ignore or filter the stimuli.

Operation Desert Storm (the U.S. offensive to counteract Iraq's invasion of Kuwait) began on January 17, 1991. The television brought moment-to-moment coverage of the war to our living room. I found it hard not to watch. We had only one television, which was situated in the living room. If I wanted to be with Ted, who spent much of his free time in front of the television set viewing the news, then I had to sit in the living room. Even if I kept my eyes on a knitting project, I could not escape the sights and sounds of the war. At my weekly appointment with Dr. Judy Shedd, she took one look at me and declared I had the classic symptoms of battle fatigue. She ruled the living room out of bounds.

Shopping also overstimulated my brain. A trip to the pharmacy or the grocery became a major undertaking requiring two or three times longer than in the past. Though I carefully followed a written list, I had to go through a laborious process just to determine which brand among many I should select for each item. For me, shopping had the same dizzying effect that attending a carnival would have posed. The many choices and products and the other shoppers—like neon lights and crowds at a carnival—utterly drained me of energy. The overstimulation exhausted me.

Sometimes, while puzzling over a purchase in a store, I heard young mothers lose patience with toddlers who asked repeatedly for a well-displayed toy. I never interrupted the dialogue between parent and child, but I often wished to tell the parent that the myriad of offerings resembled a frenetic circus to the child. I doubted that our brains were ever designed to absorb such constant stimulation.

I was grateful that my stepmother, Betty, often took me grocery shopping and patiently guided me through the marketing maze that accosted me the moment I stepped into a store. It was a tiring and often challenging experience, though not as exhausting if she was with me. Her humor also helped me to cope.

For other purchases I used mail-order services. Ted had a standing joke that I was the only one he knew who was on a first-name basis with our local UPS driver.

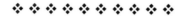

*Medical Description:*

Though frontal lobe damage interfered with the decision-making process, most of my shopping difficulties arose from injury to the temporal lobe. This caused me to become distracted by what I saw and heard and led to my difficulty in identifying and categorizing objects. When faced with multiple choices—as in a store—a shopper must go through extensive evaluation during the decision-making process of determining which item to purchase. As children grow, the process that allows them to evaluate and put things into categories develops as the brain develops. After a traumatic brain injury, a person has to relearn this evaluation process. Without such skills, shoppers might become easy targets of scammers or prone to unwise purchases. As I struggled to select the best choices among the many products for sale, I relied on the truth-in-labeling disclosures on various goods. "If my problems came to me properly labeled," I quipped, "I wouldn't have any problems at all."

# 15

# In Touch With
# My Own Pain

AFTER THE ACCIDENT, watching a movie or attending a concert or a play presented me with a new dilemma. Ted took me to a matinee, a touching drama that he thought I would enjoy, followed by a quiet dinner somewhere, only to find me dabbing my tears all through the meal. For days afterward, I was unaccountably sad. Telling myself the story was fictional provided no solace. I felt real sadness, and that emotion lingered long after I had viewed the movie. Even worse, caught in the mood the movie had stimulated, I sometimes overreacted to a seemingly innocuous situation at home.

In January 1991 while Guy was home on semester break from the University of Maine, he and I attended Spike Lee's *Do The Right Thing*. After returning home, we had a minor disagreement, the content of which neither of us recalls now. But Guy remembered my response was emotional, quite out of character for the old me. During the discussion, I quoted an inflammatory line from the movie. In fact I mimicked several lines from the movie, completely unaware of the inappropriateness of my response. It was clear to Guy that I was not acting normally.

Becoming in touch with my own pain was an important development. I soon realized I had a significant amount of internal stress that I had never acknowledged. While I had concentrated on hearing other people's pain, I had never listened to the crying of my own inner voice.

When I asked Dr. Shedd how she would have described me before the accident, she used the word *superfunctioning*. Before the accident I had tried so hard to see a situation from other people's point of view that I often shared their burdens while suppressing my own views and needs. Now I literally felt their pain. When I heard a person say unkind or malicious words about someone else, stabbing pains shot through my head. I felt as if my skull were in a vise. At times the sensation was so violent it made me want to shriek in pain.

The pain did not ease until I developed the courage to confront the speaker and say, "I find your opinion hurtful" or "I think you are being unfair" or "It hurts me to hear you say that." I had to learn to give voice to my pain or sadness in order for the pain in my head to go away.

At my six-month examination, Dr. Joseph Corbett, my neurosurgeon, said the pain likely served as a warning sign of seizures. I had taken the antiseizure medication Dilantin for a short time and had not developed seizures, but I certainly had several severe headaches.

My stepdaughter Deborah described me as someone who had retreated within myself after the accident. She recalled that I seemed to be a shell of my former self, even dressing in drabber clothes, as I spent my days struggling to gain a grip on a world that seemed foreign. Instead of the lively, self-confident woman who faced life with zest, I had become a subservient person who simply "went along" like a shadow.

Dori, another stepdaughter, recalled that she and her sisters had been surprised to hear me say a few tactless words about someone. They had never known me to use such thoughtless language in the past.

I learned that emotions typically tend to be very close to the surface in someone with frontal lobe damage. One cries easily or says exactly what is on one's mind without editing the words first. Relearning the social skill of tact takes time.

While before the accident I had often acted spontaneously, after the accident my reactions became instantaneous. I felt driven to act or reply immediately, worried that if I delayed, I would forget what I had to say or do. Since I had always been a responsible person, the fear of not meeting a duty led me to act quickly, sometimes without thinking.

Until my vision improved in early 1992 and I was able to undertake projects that involved several different tasks, planning and implementing such activities (baking a cake, even from a cake mix) remained difficult. Once I mastered that particular challenge, I became able to jot down reminders of the chores and other activities I needed to do. Only then did I become less driven to stop everything and address an interruption immediately.

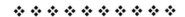

*In Retrospect:*

Learning to give voice to my own pain was perhaps one of the most valuable lessons I gained from my accident. As a parent, I had given my children a chance to tell their side of the story when a disagreement arose between them. Each voice was heard. This proved to be a successful approach to conflict resolution. However, when it came to voicing my own views, I was a failure. I had spent a lifetime trying to see things from the other person's perspective and serving as everyone else's advocate. Yet I had broken the Golden Rule that counsels us all to love our neighbor as ourselves because I had failed to love myself.

Attending monthly meetings with Roy Fairfield's writers group, gaining mastery of multitasked projects, and listening to my own inner voice became critical steps in my recovery. Keeping a journal and writing family stories also helped develop clear thinking and healthful introspection.

# 16

# Finding a Sacred Center

I DEVELOPED MANY coping skills in my recovery process. The first, and perhaps most important, had to do with keeping a journal. For years I had risen early in the morning, made a pot of coffee, and spent time in quiet meditation, reflection, prayer, and writing. It was a way to track my days, allow space for critical thinking, and proceed through life with positive intentions. I believed that taking time to evaluate life reduced the number of mistakes made.

I believed that if we did not learn from difficult circumstances, we might be doomed to a repeat performance until we finally caught on to the truth of the matter. Though I had never seen a religious theorist espouse the thought, life itself seemed to prove out the possibility. Consequently, I offered up a constant prayer, "Lord, what would You have me learn from this?" and "Lord, keep me teachable."

One morning during one of my most discouraging times, I read Psalm 90, verse 12. "So teach us to number our days, that we may apply our hearts to wisdom." Something about that verse startled me. I looked at it again. The verse did not say to number our years, our decades, our months, or our weeks. It said *days*.

I thought about that, and I realized immediately that I could free myself from so many painful expectations. I calculated my age in days (not years, months, or weeks). Then I calculated the number of days since the accident. I wrote both numbers in my journal next to the day's date.

On January 8, 1991, I was fifteen thousand, two hundred, and fifty days old, and one hundred and forty-seven days had passed since the accident. I had absolutely no preconceived ideas about how someone who was 15,250 days old ought to act, or what that person should be capable of doing. On the other hand, I had definite ideas about how someone forty-one years old ought to act, and what she ought to be able to accomplish. And when I realized that the accident that had nearly ended my life had occurred only 147 days ago, I became much more forgiving of my own failings.

With that one simple act of recalculating my longevity in days, I started to redefine how I looked at myself.

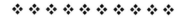

*In Retrospect:*

Reframing how I viewed myself was one of the kindest gifts I had ever given myself. This simple act became the key to parenting myself successfully and creating a sacred space from which to draw resolution and serenity. I would have allowed someone else innumerable chances to succeed. I had to learn to do the same for myself. The renumbering of my days provided the fresh perspective I needed to take each new day, each new task, and each new opportunity as a living-in-the-moment occasion. I knew full well that each new moment was a gift that had almost slipped from my hand. I could not justify squandering my energy and emotions on frustration over my failings. When I realized so few days had elapsed since the accident and each moment was a tenuous treasure, I began to forgive myself for being less than competent and not grasping former skills easily.

# 17

# Creating a Sacred Garden

I USUALLY AROSE earlier than Ted. I made coffee, then snuggled in my comfortable rocking chair in the lower den for my meditative time. My gray cat, Shadow, was my faithful companion. Together we greeted the day and peered out at the panorama of wildlife beyond the oversized bay window. Sometimes I stoked the wood fire in the Franklin stove and settled back into my quiet reverie, undisturbed in this remote corner of the house. Some would describe our backyard as *au naturel* with little lawn to maintain close to the house. It was there I decided to create a place that invited birds, butterflies, and other small creatures.

In the fall of 1990 I set bird feeders about six feet beyond the window and was rewarded almost instantly by beautiful visitors. As fall merged with winter, seed catalogs enticed me with their images, and I began to plan for a small flower and fruit garden in this area of the backyard. The next spring I planted pink cosmos, purple petunias, and white geraniums near the bird feeders. Throughout the summer I carefully tended this small patch of soil. Measuring only about 2 feet by 6 feet, it produced bursts of color and drew more feathered friends to the birdbath in the center of the plot.

Relishing my small but tangible success, I planted spring-flowering bulbs of daffodils and tulips the following September. Winter came, and the birds, mostly chickadees and blue jays, remained faithful visitors. Seed catalogs again brought their lush imagery, and I began to envision an enlarged garden that would nestle up behind the two-car garage attached to the house.

In the spring of 1992 I ordered a load of loam. Little did I realize how much loam would be delivered! The rich, dark soil filled a huge space next to the garage. The loam pile lay about fifteen feet from the garden site on relatively flat land. Since the garden had been my idea, I figured I would be the one to spread the loam.

"Sure I can do it," I said confidently. I had made quite an improvement in the year and half since the accident and thought the exercise would be good for me.

The work did not go easily. I struggled with each wheelbarrow load. While I sometimes fumed silently that no one offered to share the burden, I never asked for help. I remembered my friend Alma Field, who had struggled to achieve competence after her stroke, and I knew it was important therapy for me to be able to do the work myself. Other people did not need the therapy, I did.

In the beginning, simply shoveling loam from the pile into the wheelbarrow threw me off balance. Pushing the wheelbarrow and depositing the soil on the new garden bed exhausted me. Fortunately, my garden was small. Eventually, Guy and Adam redistributed what remained of the load to another part of the backyard. But the small backyard garden beyond my window blossomed as a result of my efforts alone. It became an important haven for me, where I could find serenity and

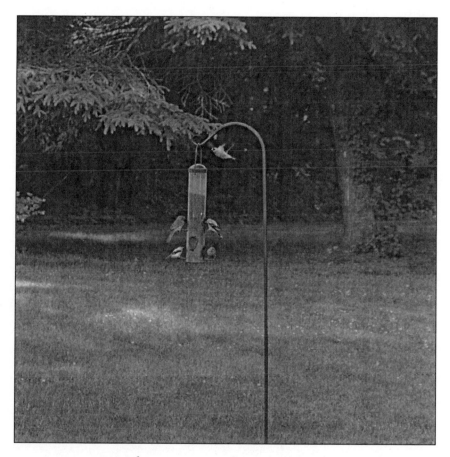

encouragement when aspects of my recovery seemed to proceed far too slowly.

I planted purple, yellow, and blue pansies; red, white, and
salmon geraniums; pink, orange, and white daylilies; cosmos in
shades of hot pink; and vibrant red bee balm; and bordered
it all with gold and apricot marigolds and nasturtiums. It created a vibrant rainbow of colors. I collected wild violets from
the lawn and transplanted them into a nearby raised flower bed.
Then I watched the butterflies come.

The visual symphony I had created in cooperation with

Mother Nature soothed me. My spirit quieted and became enraptured as I gazed at the interplay of bird, butterfly, and petal. Beautiful birds rewarded me with their presence and cheerful chattering as soon as I filled the feeders. I thoroughly enjoyed the playful antics of the chipmunks and squirrels and watched intently the society of wildlife when a maimed squirrel came to feed. Amazingly, the other creatures always seemed to make room for this one wounded being.

Each day I watched for the little gray squirrel, somewhat smaller than the others and with an amputated tail and shortened back leg, as he made his way to the bird feeder. Respectfully (or so it seemed to me), the other squirrels and birds held back to allow him room. After the wounded creature had eaten his fill, the chatter and busyness about the feeder resumed. Life went on as usual. And yet, for me, it was different. I felt confirmed and quietly thrilled.

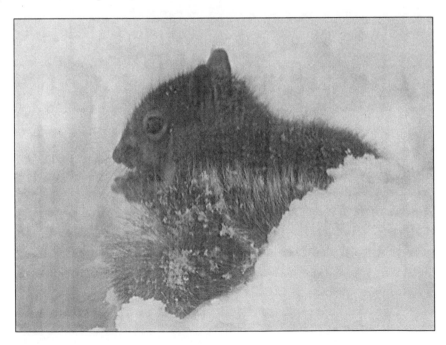

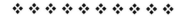

*In Retrospect:*

Focusing on creating a world that was safe for the most fragile creatures gave me hope that I, too, would find a place in the world where I would be safe in my fragility. The garden and bird sanctuary brought almost immediate rewards and became an important contribution to my recovery, where progress was anything but instantaneous. Planting flowers and watching them grow, putting up feeders and seeing the birds respond fed my soul and gave me patience to continue with the slow progress toward recovery.

The garden also brought me visual beauty, not the clutter and disorder that, for me, represented my sometimes cluttered and disordered mind. As I viewed the garden's soothing loveliness, my mind became soothed, too. The fact that I had created something beautiful and soothing outside told me that perhaps I could re-create something lovely inside. The plot of ground outside my window became my genesis garden, reminding me that God created order out of chaos, and it was good.

# Section IV

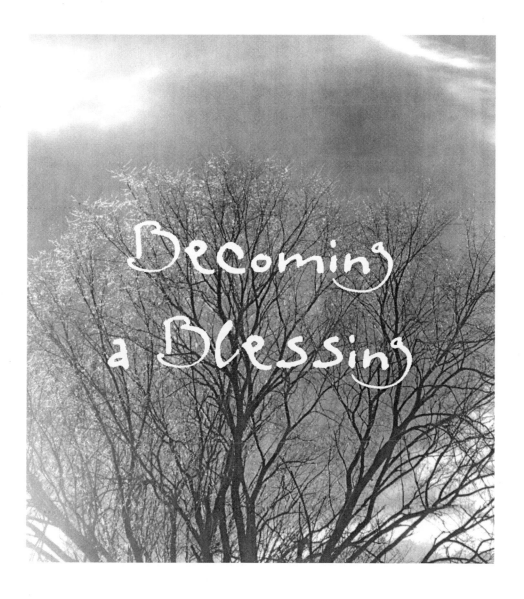

Becoming a Blessing

# The Primal Chord

As a participant
In my own evolution,
    Concurrently I stretch
        Back to my roots,
        And forward to my calling—
Ever being tuned
By the tension of the pull,
    Backward
        And onward,
        All at once.
Trying to pluck
The truest chord—
    To denote
        With integrity,
        Who I am.

EAC/1993

# 18

# Repacking Bags for Life

I MAY NEVER RIDE a bike again; then again, I may. But at least I know I can if I want to. I do not have to be plagued by fear, but I can choose to use good judgment. I give myself permission to say, simply, "No."

I have developed a variety of coping skills, some of which I adapted from the Learning Disability Association's tips on how to improve the quality of life for those with attention deficit hyperactivity disorder or dyslexia.

For concentration problems:
1. Focus on the speaker's face—this helps counteract my hearing loss as well as improving concentration.
2. Do one thing at a time, but maintain a running list of other things that need to be done. Politely refuse to be distracted unless it is an emergency.
3. Control noise and outside stimuli.
4. Rest when needed, and don't feel guilty about it.

For organizational problems:
1. Post a calendar on the wall. Mark every appointment including time and phone reference.
2. Look at the calendar each day.
3. Keep a corresponding calendar in my purse and update it daily.
4. Make a to-do list each night. Check it off throughout the day. Keep it current.

Bike helmets are mandatory in my family. It is the cheapest insurance possible. Even if there's nothing worth saving in your head, I tell family members, you will have lost nothing by wearing a helmet!

I always followed my own rules for living while on the road to recovery:
1. Get dressed every day—never stay in pajamas past the time for morning coffee.
2. Take naps—a way to respect the body's needs during recovery.
3. Leave yourself notes—keep them in a pocket to refer to easily.
4. Try to do something nice for someone else daily.
5. Keep a daily journal—if only to clarify thoughts.
6. Take high-potency vitamins under doctor's guidance and eat healthy foods.
7. Find at least one thing to be thankful for every day.

Like my friend Linda, I believe I am in many ways at 110 percent. Although I cannot and perhaps never will be able to perform some activities I could have accomplished easily before my accident, I have gained wisdom and gratitude for each new day. I have been blessed with fine doctors, particularly Dr. Judy Shedd; a loving family; and supportive friends. My journey of healing became, in many respects, an inward odyssey that manifested itself in outward healing. I now know myself far better than I ever thought I needed to, and I have utter respect for the messages my body sends me.

I have learned to apply these simple truths as I repack my bags for life. Fear is a terrible burden to carry, weighing heavier each time the bag is lifted; but foolishness is an even heavier burden, because it often hurts others as well. My recovery has taught me to weigh decisions carefully before taking action. I now have the patience to wait and consider. I do not think I have to solve every problem, nor do I have to meet every responsibility that is within my sight. Discernment considerably lightens my load.

A banner that hangs in the sanctuary of my church speaks to me. It says, "You have been Blessed, now go and be a Blessing." Undeniably, we all have choices in our lives. I have chosen to try to be a blessing.

# 19

# Left Brain, Right Brain, No Brain

THERE IS NO CURE FOR TRAUMATIC BRAIN INJURY. Dead brain cells never become alive again. That does not mean a person with TBI cannot contribute in a vital way to the family or community. It merely means the contributions will be different from those the person once imagined. Most people pursue multiple careers in a lifespan; TBI often forces those changes on an individual. I have had to discard old agendas and dreams and learn to see the possibilities in new horizons.

Through steady work, I have been able to develop learning skills and new ways of doing old jobs. Today, in the year 2009, I use my left hand to do many activities, though I still consider myself primarily right-handed. After hours of practice, I can perform many activities almost automatically. I knit with reasonable ease, although I tend to choose simpler patterns than I used before the accident. I paint with watercolors, pastels, and mixed media. I am proficient in the kitchen and can organize and execute challenging projects. I set up a library at a local county jail; yet whenever I have to reshelve books, I always pause and quietly recite the children's alphabet rhyme before placing the book in its proper spot. I still have to recheck mathematical calculations with a calculator and double-check to ensure I have copied numbers accurately. Weeding our hillside garden makes me dizzy. I carefully view a crowded room to determine the best location to accommodate my hearing problems. I often prefer to avoid noisy locales and generally limit phone conversations. I still catch myself stepping into traffic without looking both ways. I am selective about the movies I view and the music I listen to because of the way they affect me. I watch in-depth news programs that handle topics in a thoughtful, civilized manner and avoid the emotional diatribes of "news jockeys" and talk radio commentators that leave me distracted and distraught.

When I look in a mirror, I still see telltale scars from lacerations and an odd bump on my forehead where a monitoring tube was inserted into my skull. The mirror reminds me that each day is a gift.

My brain gives me a gentle, sometimes not so gentle, warning when I become overtired. It's like a whisper reminding me, "You are dealing with a damaged organ and need to rest now." Sometimes my brain puts the brakes on, and I simply cannot think. It says to me, "Sorry, gone on vacation."

I sleep well. If I do not retire by ten P.M., I often feel the onset of a headache—a signal that it is bedtime. Before the accident I often suffered from insomnia. It has never been a problem since the accident. During the early days of my recovery, I slept soundly because I was utterly exhausted at the end of each day. Everything required so much concentration to eke out the smallest results.

I have confronted social obstacles as well as physical injuries in order to heal. Denial, my own as well as other people's, blocked my way until I dealt with it. Looking whole did not mean that I *was* whole. I might have received more understanding (even from myself!) if I had suffered broken bones instead of a broken brain. People could have identified my injury more easily if they had been able to see it. Because I looked relatively normal and could speak, people believed that I was healed. As a consequence, family and friends resisted any change in the role I had always played in their lives. No one wanted to accept the possibility that I had diminished capabilities—even if it was temporary.

As I labored through the deeper work of healing, I came to realize that even if I could no longer perform the old functions with ease as I once did, my life was still worth living. I had to face my own fears before I could truly heal. I had to confront my own embarrassment at my failings before further healing could take place. My sense of humor and my celebration of every seemingly inconsequential victory enabled me to continue on this arduous journey toward recovery.

I also had to overcome the tendency of other people, well-meaning but misguided, to take over tasks that I was trying to do. Such behavior increased my sense of incompetence. Although I valued help when I needed it, I knew that too much help would hinder my development. I was blessed with helpers who intuitively understood the difference.

For all the innovative therapy and public awareness this painful condition has engendered, the basic facts remain the same. The hard and rocky road toward recovery of a "normal" life requires the constant, difficult day-by-day work of the patient and the caregiver. Recovery does not come at the speed of the sprinter but at the steady pace of the marathon runner.

# Appendices

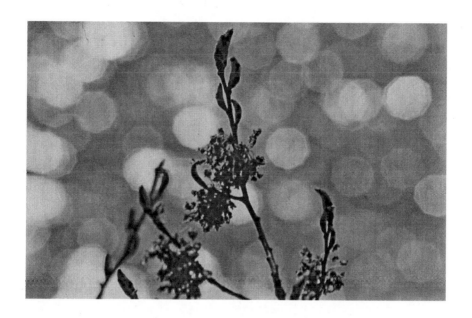

# Appendix 1

## Recovery Timeline

August 14, 1990: Bicycle accident.

August 27, 1990: Released from hospital.

March 1991: Drove car short distances in light traffic (plotted route beforehand).

Spring 1991: Created "left-handed" floral wreath. This was the first indication that new networks were developing in my brain to take over old jobs. Tackled simple knitting projects: 8-inch-square dishcloth (ten hours to complete).

August 1991: Rode a bicycle again for about 1,000 feet.
　　　Was able to cook a simple meal from scratch.

1993: Rode alone in elevator without having panic attack.

May 1994: Successfully flew alone to Spain to accompany Adam home from year's study abroad. Negotiating busy airports was challenging, but I did it!

October 1994: Successfully made way through Boston subways.

1996: Snowshoed without panic attack caused by the feeling that the world was sliding away beneath my feet.

Fall 1998: Wrote and illustrated poetry chapbook.

June 1999: Rode escalator without having panic attack.

June 2000–2001: Took art class in pastels and mixed media; finally succeeded in drawing vase that did not look lopsided.

Fall 2001: Took lessons in Nordic Hardanger embroidery. Used my right hand but followed left-handed diagrams and instructions, which I had adapted. The process took four times longer to accomplish than it would have otherwise. I was ever so grateful for my patient instructor.

# Appendix 2

## The Brain

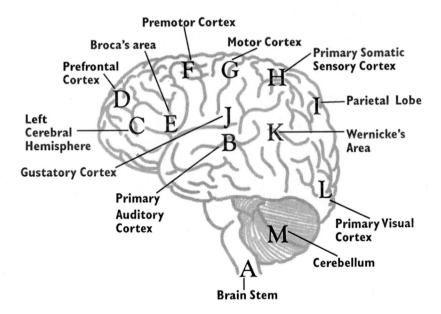

Premotor Cortex

Broca's area

Motor Cortex

Prefrontal Cortex

Primary Somatic Sensory Cortex

F  G  H

D

I — Parietal Lobe

Left Cerebral Hemisphere — C  E

J

K — Wernicke's Area

B

Gustatory Cortex

Primary Auditory Cortex

L

M

Primary Visual Cortex

A

Cerebellum

Brain Stem

# The Brain

**A  brain stem:** controls unconscious functions such as breathing and blood pressure.

**B  primary auditory cortex:** interprets quality of sound (tone, loudness).

**C  left cerebral hemisphere:** with right cerebral hemisphere, controls thought, language, and movement control. Right hemisphere controls activities performed by left side of body; left hemisphere controls those by right side of body.

**D  prefrontal cortex:** involved in planning, abstract reasoning, putting things in sequence, social behavior, concentration, personality, and mood.

**E  Broca's area:** responsible for speech.

**F  premotor cortex:** linked to complex movements, including gait.

**G  motor cortex:** controls voluntary movement.

**H  primary somatic sensory cortex:** processes sensations of touch.

**I  parietal lobe:** linked to language, writing, math, spatial relations, pain, and touch.

**J  gustatory cortex:** responsible for taste sensations.

**K  Wernicke's area:** involved in understanding and using speech.

**L  primary visual cortex:** receives visual input from the eyes.

**M  cerebellum:** controls balance and fine-motor coordination.

Source: "Atlas of the Body: The Brain—After a Stroke," AMA's Current Procedural Terminology, rev. ed. Medical Library, American Medical Association. On line at http://www.ama-assn.org/ama/pub/physician-resources/patient-education-materials/atlas-of-human-body/brain-effects-stroke.shtml

# The Brain

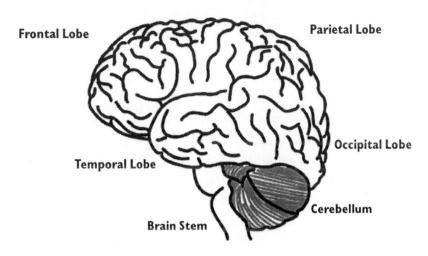

Frontal Lobe    Parietal Lobe

Occipital Lobe

Temporal Lobe

Cerebellum

Brain Stem

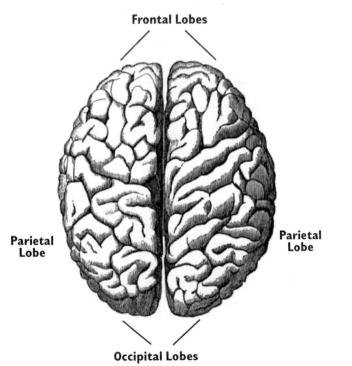

Frontal Lobes

Parietal
Lobe

Parietal
Lobe

Occipital Lobes

# Appendix 3

## Resources

**The Brain Injury Association of America** (BIAA) actively advocates for victims and families of victims. Regional and state rehabilitation centers are great sources of help. BIAA operates offices in every state in the nation. The organization's website is at www.biausa.org.

**The Defense and Veteran Brain Injury Center**, operated by and for the military, has a website at www.DVBIC.org. Because TBI is considered the "signature injury" of veterans of the Iraq and Afghanistan wars, the military has become proactive in caring for veterans with TBI. The organization's online newsletter, *Brainwaves*, features up-to-date articles and contact information for veterans.

**BrainSource**, an informational website operated by neuropsychologist Dennis P. Swiercinsky, Ph.D., offers useful facts about TBI. The website can be found at www.brainsource.com. According to the BIAA, someone sustains a traumatic brain injury every fifteen seconds in America. Each year 1.4 million Americans suffer a traumatic brain injury, and 126,000 are permanently disabled annually. In addition, an estimated 320,000 U.S. veterans of the Iraq and Afghanistan wars have TBI.

**Judy Hetzler Shedd, D.O.**, uses a homeopathic and osteopathic approach to treating TBI, a method that proved successful for me. Her website is at www.JudyShedd.com.

**Maine Neurorehabilitation Facilities**: Currently in Maine there are numerous facilities specific to neuro/ABI/TBI treatment. Among them:

BANGOR

Acadia Hospital, 268 Stillwater Avenue, Bangor, ME 04401 (207) 973-6100 or (800) 640-1211

BREWER

Maine Center for Integrated Rehabilitation (private outpatient treatment program), Twin City Plaza, 248 State St., Brewer, ME, 04412, (207) 989-2034; facilities also located in Fairfield and Rockland

KENNEBUNK

RiverRidge Rehabilitation (inpatient, long-term residential care and outpatient services), 3 Brazier Lane, Kennebunk, ME, 04043, (207) 985-3030

LEWISTON

Westside Neurorehabilitation Services (outpatient/day treatment), 618 Main Street, Lewiston, ME 04240, (207) 795-6110 V/TTY, (800) 352-9547 toll-free

PORTLAND

Bayside Neurorehabilitation Services (outpatient/day treatment), 26 Portland Street, Portland, ME 04101, (207) 761-8402 V/TTY, (800) 341-4516 toll-free

New England Rehabilitation Hospital (acute inpatient and outpatient), 335 Brighton Avenue, Portland, ME 04102, Referral Services: (207) 662-8584, Admissions Office: (207) 662-8584, Outpatient Center: (207) 662-8377

**General services**: At various Maine hospitals, including:

Goodall Hospital (outpatient treatment), 25 June Street, Sanford, ME 04073, (207) 324-4310

Maine Medical Center—Barbara Bush Center (children's

care), Richards Wing (acute rehabilitation with transfer to New England Rehabilitation Hospital), 22 Bramhall Street, Portland, ME 04102, (207) 662-0111

Midcoast–Central Maine Medical Center (inpatient and outpatient rehab services), 300 Main St., Lewiston, ME 04240, (207) 532-2900

York Hospital (outpatient treatment), 15 Hospital Drive, York, ME 03909, (207) 363-4321

**Veterans' Services**

**In Maine**: Centralized through the Togus VA Medical Center, 1 VA Center, Augusta, ME 04330, www.togus.va.gov. The hospital is located just outside Augusta in Chelsea, Maine, toll-free 1-877-421-8263 or (207) 623-8411. Eight community-based outpatient clinics for veterans are located throughout the state. They are located in Bangor, Calais, Caribou, Fort Kent, Houlton, Lincoln, Rumford, and Saco. Mental health clinics for veterans operate in Bangor and Portland.

**Throughout the United States**: A little-known program called the Aid and Attendance Benefit provides financial assistance to eligible veterans and spouses to pay for a health-care provider after injury. The benefit covers assisted-living care either in a nursing home or in the recipient's own home. It may also pay the spouse for providing care if he or she has to leave work to care for the injured person. Contact the VA or Veteran Aid.org for more details about the program.

More information on veterans services can also be found at www.maineveteranshomes.org (Maine) and www.va.gov (U.S.). The primary contact and referral information for veterans who think they may suffer from ABI/TBI is through Defense and Veteran Brain Injury Center, www.DVBIC.org, (800)870-9244.

# Bibliography

Bolen, Jean Shinoda. *Goddesses in Every Woman.* New York: Harper & Row, 1984. This was the perfect book to help me gain self-acceptance when I was struggling with my own identity.

Borysenko, Joyce. *Guilt is the Teacher, Love is the Lesson.* New York: Warner Books Inc, 1990.

———. *Minding the Body, Mending the Mind.* New York: Bantam Books Inc., 1988. Based on the programs of the Mind/Body Clinic at New England Deaconess Hospital, these two books gave me tools for relaxation using an holistic approach to deal with pain and confusion in the healing process.

Cousins, Norman. *Anatomy of an Illness.* New York: Bantam Books, 1979. It was so encouraging to read of Cousins's success in curing himself as I teamed up with my physicians on my own journey to recovery.

Ealy, C. Diane. *The Woman's Book of Creativity.* Hillsboro, OR: Beyond Woods Pub., 1995. This was the first time I realized women's mind processes are different from men's.

Fairfield, Roy P. *Person-Centered Graduate Education.* New York: Prometheus Books, 1977. This book details a style of learning appropriate for adults that became the basis for the Union Graduate School's pioneering work with independent learners.

Hoffman, Edward. *The Right to be Human: A Biography of Abraham Maslow.* Los Angeles, CA: Jeremy P. Tarcher Inc., 1988. Hoffman does a wonderful job of describing the man who led the self-actualization movement.

Ledoux, Denis. *Turning Memories into Memoirs: A Handbook for Writing Lifestories.* Lisbon Falls, ME: Soleil Press, 1993. Ledoux's style of drawing out the life story each has within provides a superb model for making sense of one's life.

Le Poncin, Monique. *Brain Fitness.* Trans. by Lowell Bair. New York: Random House, 1990. In her work for the French National Institute for Research on the Prevention of Cerebral Aging, Le Poncin created a series of simple exercises designed to encourage new links in the brain. Initially these exercises were difficult for me, but they became easier as I went through them.

*The New King James Version of the Holy Bible.* Pasadena, CA: Thomas Nelson Inc., 1988. From this ancient and sacred collection, I drew encouragement from the *Book of Psalms* in particular. The verses were both subtle and raw, portraying the ordeal of a struggling people trying to make sense of their world. *Proverbs*, also extraordinarily helpful, drew me back to timeless basics. *Philippians* guided me in finding joy in dark places.

Sarton, May. *After the Stroke, A Journal.* New York: W.W. Norton & Co., 1988. Sarton's tenacity in journaling her recovery after her stroke gave me encouragement and provided dignity to the healing process.

Sinetar, Marsha. *Elegant Choices, Healing Choices.* Mahwah, NJ: Paulist Press, 1988. A wise and wonderful book that encourages living in a way that builds self-esteem.

Tillich, Paul. *The Courage to Be.* 2nd Ed. New Haven, CT: Yale University Press, 1952. Tillich helped me put anxiety in perspective. His depth, scope, and personal history provided valuable insights.

Vincent, Marilyn C. and Margaret Merrion. "The Musical Mind Considered: A New Frontier," *Design for Arts in Education.* Sept/Oct. 1990: 11–18. This is the first article that gave me hope about stimulating creativity in the brain by listening to good music.

Willard, Frank H. and Daniel P. Perl. *Medical Neuroanatomy: a*

*Problem-Oriented Manual with Annotated Atlas.* Philadelphia, PA: J.B. Lippincott Co., 1993. This is a medical textbook that can be read by laymen. I borrowed it from my doctor to help gain insight into what was happening in my head.

Woodruff, Lee. "Can Brains Be Saved?" *Parade*, July 12, 2009. An updated report on the progress of TBI treatment by the wife of Bob Woodruff, the ABC reporter who suffered from TBI while in Iraq.

Wycoff, Joyce. *Mindmapping.* New York: Berkley Books, 1991. This was an encouraging volume. It was a good book to read a second time after a one-year break. Wycoff offers many strategies to develop creative approaches to problems.

**Books written by victims of TBI:**

Mandrell, Barbara, George Vecsey. *Get to the Heart.* New York: Bantam Books, 1990. This was a bit confusing the first time I read it. Going back a second time, I realized it was written as a memoir for her many fans to enjoy—but it does give encouragement on being able to resume one's previous work after TBI.

Osborn, Claudia L. *Over my Head.* Kansas City: Andrews McMeel Pub., 1998. Dr. Osborn was injured in a bicycle accident and chronicles her recovery in an honest way that any victim of TBI can connect with. Because of her medical background, she had access to more aids than were available to me, but her struggles remained much the same as those of any TBI victim.

Woodruff, Lee and Bob Woodruff. *In an Instant.* New York: Random House, 2007. Website at www.ReMind.org. Bob Woodruff was injured in Iraq while covering the war for ABC. This is an honest and courageous account of his ordeal as well as the whole family's struggle during his recovery process.

Printed in the United States
221745BV00004B/1/P

9 781892 168139